LEPTOMENINGEAL METASTASES

Cancer Treatment and Research
Steven T. Rosen, M.D., *Series Editor*

Sugarbaker, P. (ed): *Peritoneal Carcinomatosis: Principles of Management.* 1995. ISBN 0-7923-3727-1.
Dickson, R.B., Lippman, M.E. (eds.): *Mammary Tumor Cell Cycle, Differentiation and Metastasis.* 1995. ISBN 0-7923-3905-3.
Freireich, E.J, Kantarjian, H.(eds):*Molecular Genetics and Therapy of Leukemia.* 1995. ISBN 0-7923-3912-6.
Cabanillas, F., Rodriguez, M.A.(eds): *Advances in Lymphoma Research.* 1996. ISBN 0-7923-3929-0.
Miller, A.B. (ed.): *Advances in Cancer Screening.* 1996. ISBN 0-7923-4019-1.
Hait , W.N. (ed.): *Drug Resistance.* 1996. ISBN 0-7923-4022-1.
Pienta, K.J. (ed.): *Diagnosis and Treatment of Genitourinary Malignancies.* 1996. ISBN 0-7923-4164-3.
Arnold, A.J. (ed.): *Endocrine Neoplasms.* 1997. ISBN 0-7923-4354-9.
Pollock, R.E. (ed.): *Surgical Oncology.* 1997. ISBN 0-7923-9900-5.
Verweij, J., Pinedo, H.M., Suit, H.D. (eds): *Soft Tissue Sarcomas: Present Achievements and Future Prospects.* 1997. ISBN 0-7923-9913-7.
Walterhouse, D.O., Cohn, S. L. (eds.): *Diagnostic and Therapeutic Advances in Pediatric Oncology.* 1997. ISBN 0-7923-9978-1.
Mittal, B.B., Purdy, J.A., Ang, K.K. (eds): *Radiation Therapy.* 1998. ISBN 0-7923-9981-1.
Foon, K.A., Muss, H.B. (eds): *Biological and Hormonal Therapies of Cancer.* 1998. ISBN 0-7923-9997-8.
Ozols, R.F. (ed.): *Gynecologic Oncology.* 1998. ISBN 0-7923-8070-3.
Noskin, G. A. (ed.): *Management of Infectious Complications in Cancer Patients.* 1998. ISBN 0-7923-8150-5.
Bennett, C. L. (ed.): *Cancer Policy.* 1998. ISBN 0-7923-8203-X.
Benson, A. B. (ed.): *Gastrointestinal Oncology.* 1998. ISBN 0-7923-8205-6.
Tallman, M.S., Gordon, L.I. (eds): *Diagnostic and Therapeutic Advances in Hematologic Malignancies.* 1998. ISBN 0-7923-8206-4.
von Gunten, C.F. (ed): *Palliative Care and Rehabilitation of Cancer Patients.* 1999. ISBN 0-7923-8525-X
Burt, R.K., Brush, M.M. (eds): *Advances in Allogeneic Hematopoietic Stem Cell Transplantation.* 1999. ISBN 0-7923-7714-1.
Angelos, P. (ed.): *Ethical Issues in Cancer Patient Care* 2000. ISBN 0-7923-7726-5.
Gradishar, W.J., Wood, W.C. (eds): *Advances in Breast Cancer Management.* 2000. ISBN 0-7923-7890-3.
Sparano, Joseph A. (ed.): *HIV & HTLV-I Associated Malignancies.* 2001. ISBN 0-7923-7220-4.
Ettinger, David S. (ed.): *Thoracic Oncology.* 2001. ISBN 0-7923-7248-4.
Bergan, Raymond C. (ed.): *Cancer Chemoprev*ention. 2001. ISBN 0-7923-7259-X.
Raza, A., Mundle, S.D. (eds): *Myelodysplastic Syndromes & Secondary Acute Myelogenous Leukemia* 2001. ISBN: 0-7923-7396.
Talamonti, Mark S. (ed.): *Liver Directed Therapy for Primary and Metastatic Liver Tumors.* 2001. ISBN 0-7923-7523-8.
Stack, M.S., Fishman, D.A. (eds): *Ovarian Cancer.* 2001. ISBN 0-7923-7530-0.
Bashey, A., Ball, E.D. (eds): *Non-Myeloablative Allogeneic Transplantation.* 2002. ISBN 0-7923-7646-3.
Leong, Stanley P.L. (ed.): *Atlas of Selective Sentinel Lymphadenectomy for Melanoma, Breast Cancer and Colon Cancer.* 2002. ISBN 1-4020-7013-6.
Andersson , B., Murray D. (eds): *Clinically Relevant Resistance in Cancer Chemotherapy.* 2002. ISBN 1-4020-7200-7.
Beam, C. (ed.): *Biostatistical Applications in Cancer Research.* 2002. ISBN 1-4020-7226-0.
Brockstein, B., Masters, G. (eds): *Head and Neck Cancer.* 2003. ISBN 1-4020-7336-4.
Frank, D.A. (ed.): *Signal Transduction in Cancer.* 2003. ISBN 1-4020-7340-2.
Figlin, Robert A. (ed.): *Kidney Cancer.* 2003. ISBN 1-4020-7457-3.
Kirsch, Matthias; Black, Peter McL. (ed.): *Angiogenesis in Brain Tumors.* 2003. ISBN 1-4020-7704-1.
Keller, E.T., Chung, L.W.K. (eds): *The Biology of Skeletal Metastases.* 2004. ISBN 1-4020-7749-1.
Kumar, Rakesh (ed.): *Molecular Targeting and Signal Transduction.* 2004. ISBN 1-4020-7822-6.
Verweij, J., Pinedo, H.M. (eds): *Targeting Treatment of Soft Tissue Sarcomas.* 2004. ISBN 1-4020-7808-0.
Finn, W.G., Peterson, L.C. (eds.): *Hematopathology in Oncology.* 2004. ISBN 1-4020-7919-2.
Farid, N., (ed): *Molecular Basis of Thyroid Cancer.* 2004. ISBN 1-4020-8106-5.
Khleif, S., (ed): *Tumor Immunology and Cancer* Vaccines. 2004. ISBN 1-4020-8119-7.
Balducci, L., Extermann, M. (eds.): *Biological Basis of Geriatric Oncology.* 2004. ISBN
Abrey, L.E., Chamberlain, M.C., Engelhard, H.H. (eds.): *Leptomeningeal Metastases.* 2005. ISBN 0-387-24198-
Leong, Stanley P.L., Kitagawa, Y., Kitajima, M. (eds.): *Selective Sentinel Lymphadenectomy for Human Solid Cancer* 2005. ISBN 0-387-23603-1

LEPTOMENINGEAL METASTASES

edited by

LAUREN E. ABREY, M.D.
Department of Neurology
Memorial Sloan-Kettering Cancer Center
New York, New York 10021

MARC C. CHAMBERLAIN, M.D.
Department of Neurology
University of Southern California
Norris Comprehensive Cancer Center and Hospital
Los Angeles, California

and

HERBERT H. ENGELHARD, M.D., PH.D.
Departments of Neurosurgery, Bioengineering and Molecular Genetics
University of Illinois at Chicago
Chicago, Illinois

Springer

Lauren E. Abrey, MD
Department of Neurology
Memorial Sloan-Kettering Cancer Center
1275 York Avenue
New York, NY 10021

Herbert H. Engelhard, MD, PhD
Departments of Neurosurgery,
Bioengineering & Molecular Genetics
University of Illinois at Chicago
Chicago, IL 60612

Marc C. Chamberlain, MD
Department of Neurology
University of Southern California
Norris Comprehensive Cancer Center and Hospital
Los Angeles, CA 90033

Leptomeningeal Metastases

Library of Congress Cataloging-in-Publication Data

A C.I.P. Catalogue record for this book is available
from the Library of Congress.

ISBN 0-387-24198-1 e-ISBN 0-387-24199-X Printed on acid-free paper.

Printed in the United States of America.

9 8 7 6 5 4 3 2 1 SPIN 11048770

springeronline.com

Contents

INTRODUCTION

Leptomeningeal metastases are an increasingly important complication of systemic malignancy. Historically, leptomeningeal dissemination was detected in the setting of widespread systemic tumor progression and heralded the terminal phase of a patient's tumor. However, as current solid tumor therapies have improved, it is becoming more common to encounter isolated leptomeningeal progression in a patient with a quiescent systemic tumor. Furthermore, as cancer patients are surviving longer, the incidence of leptomeningeal metastases appears to be increasing, particularly in solid tumor types not previously associated with leptomeningeal spread such as ovarian and colorectal cancer. Therefore, it is critical to have a complete understanding of the disease process and therapeutic options in order to optimize the management of patients with leptomeningeal tumor. Select patients who are managed aggressively can have prolonged survival with preservation of neurologic function and quality of life.

Optimal management of leptomeningeal metastasis requires a multi-disciplinary approach. This book draws on the expertise of neurosurgeons, medical oncologists, neurologists, neuro-oncologists, pediatric oncologists and radiation oncologists. As a result, this book provides an excellent overview of this disease process from the anatomy and physiology of the cerebrospinal fluid compartment to the scope and impact of this complication in specific malignancies. Current treatment options, both symptomatic and therapeutic, as well as new approaches to treatment are carefully reviewed. As it is clear that better therapies are desperately needed for this patient population, therapies in development and future research directions are the focus of the last chapter.

ACKNOWLEDGMENT

The editors are indebted to the assistance of Judith Mandel Lampron, who proofread, edited, and formatted all of the text, tables and references. Without her help, completion of this book would not have been possible.

Lauren E. Abrey, M.D.
Memorial Sloan-Kettering Cancer Center

Chapter 1

ANATOMY AND PHYSIOLOGY OF THE LEPTOMENINGES AND CSF SPACE

Neil Barshes, MD,[1] Alexis Demopoulos, MD,[2] Herbert H. Engelhard, MD, PhD[1]
[1]The University of Illinois at Chicago, Chicago, IL 60612; [2]Memorial Sloan-Kettering Cancer Center, 1275 York Avenue, New York, NY 10021

Abstract: The arachnoid membrane and pia mater are the two membranous layers that comprise the leptomeninges. Cerebrospinal fluid is made within the ventricular system by cells of the choroid plexus and ependyma. This chapter describes in detail the normal anatomic structure and physiologic interactions of the cerebrospinal fluid and leptomeningeal space that are critical to our understanding and treatment of leptomeningeal metastases.

Key words: Arachnoid; pia mater; leptomeninges; cerebrospinal fluid.

1. INTRODUCTION

The term *leptomeninges* refers to the inner two of the three membranous layers which envelop the brain: the arachnoid membrane and the pia mater. The prefix *lepto-*, denoting "fine" or "thin" in Greek, contrasts the properties of these two layers from the "thick" or *pachy*meningeal layer called the dura mater.[1]

Whereas the dura mater and pia mater have been described since the time of the Egyptians some 3000 years ago, the arachnoid mater was not clearly distinguished as a separate layer until the work of the Dutch anatomist Gerardus Blaes in 1666.[2] The term *arachnoid* was applied by the Dutch anatomist Frederick Ruysch (1638-1731), the name roughly meaning "spider-like" and referring to the web-like structure of this layer.[3] Axel Key and Gustaf Retzius[4] made a landmark contribution to the anatomy of these layers with their 1875 publication *Studien in der Anatomie des Nervensystem und des Bindegewebes.* The understanding of these layers has progressed even further with the development of electron microscopy and other modern research techniques.

2. EMBRYOLOGY OF THE LEPTOMENINGES

The leptomeninges are formed from both mesenchymal and neural crest cells, which surround the neural tube during development[5,6,7]. This formation begins at the 22 to 24 day stage of development, as the neural folds are beginning to fuse dorsally to form a tube-like structure. At this time, a thin monolayer of cells derived from the neural crest surrounds the developing neural tube. Between gestational days 24 and 40, mesenchymal cells migrate inward to surround first the developing spinal cord and soon after the developing brain. By gestational day 40 these cells are recognizable as a layer referred to as the *meninx primitiva*, or *primary meninx.*[5]

Two components form this primary meninx: a thin inner *ectomesenchyme*, which combines with the neural crest elements to form the *endomeninx*; and an external layer of ordinary mesenchyme which forms the *ectomeninx.* [8,5,7,6] The endomeninx will form the leptomeninges while the ectomeninx will form the dura mater[5,8]. Between days 34-48 the inner endomeninx becomes more loosely arranged while the outer ectomeninx becomes more compact.[5]

Between gestational days 45-55 the loosely arranged endomeninx surrounds and envelops the blood vessels which are forming on the surface of the developing brain and spinal cord.[5,9] By this stage of development the denticulate ligaments are well-formed. Cavitations within the ectomeninx also appear at this stage, initiating the development of the subarachnoid space. By gestational day 50 these spaces enlarge to form cisterns, and dural sinuses begin to develop in the ectomeninx layer.[5] The production of cerebrospinal fluid (CSF) by the *tela choroidea* is initiated in the fifth week of gestational development.[10] The pia and dura may be recognized as separate layers at approximately day 50. The arachnoid layer may not be recognizable as a separate layer until late fetal life or early postnatal life.[7]

2.1 Gross anatomy of the cerebral and spinal leptomeninges

The cerebral leptomeninges are anchored to the skull via their attachment to the dura mater.[11,5] A number of CSF cisterns in the subarachnoid space have been described.[11,1,12] A summary of important features of these cisterns is listed in Table 1.

Table 1: Major CSF cisterns and contents [adapted from [5,12]]

Cistern	Arteries	Cranial Nerves	Other
Superior cerebellopontine	AICA	V, VII-VIII	--
Inferior cerebellopontine	vertebral, PICA	IX-XII	choroid plexus, olivary eminence
prepontine cistern	basilar, AICA, SCA	VI	--
cisterna magna	PICA, PSA, choroidal	--	roots of C1, C2
Interpeduncular cistern	bifurcation of basilar, PCA, SCA, choroidal, thalamogeniculate	III	mammillary body, medial crus cerebri
crural cistern	AChorA, MedPostChorA	--	--
chiasmatic cistern	ACA	II and chiasm	hypophyseal stalk
carotid cistern	ICA, AChorA and PCommA, proximal opthalmic	--	--
Sylvian	MCA	--	insular gyri
lamina terminalis cistern	ACA, ACommA, Heubner's, hypothalamic, fronto-orbital	--	--
Quadrigeminal cistern	post pericallosal, SCA (3rd portion)	IV	
ambient cistern	PCA, SCA, quadrigeminal	IV	lateral crus cerebri

Abbreviations: A1 /A2= 1st/2nd segment of Anterior Cerebral Artery; ACA= Anterior Cerebral Artery; AChorA= Anterior Choroidal Artery; ACommA= Anterior Communicating Artery; ACommV= Anterior Communicating Vein; AICA= Anterior Inferior Cerebellar Artery; ICA= Internal Carotid Artery; MCA= Middle Cerebral Artery; MCV= Middle Cerebral Vein; MedPostChorA= Medial Posterior Choroidal Vein; P1-P3= 1st through 3rd segments of Posterior Cerebral Artery; PCA= Posterior Cerebral Artery; PCommA= Posterior Communicating Artery; PICA= Posterior Inferior Cerebellar Artery; PSA= Posterior Spinal Artery; SCA= Superior Cerebral Artery.

The arrangement of the layers of the spinal leptomeninges differs significantly from that of the cerebral leptomeninges because of the presence of an actual epidural space in the spine. The epidural space is found caudal to the attachment of the dura to the foramen magnum[13] and contains the epidural veins, lymphatics, and adipose tissue.[5]

Attachment of the pia to the arachnoid in the spine is not accomplished by the random arrangement of arachnoid trabeculae, as in the cranium. Rather, there is a regular arrangement of septae. The *longitudinal midline dorsal septum* is one of these septae. It is a condensation of arachnoid, which extends from the dorsal midline arachnoid, encloses the mid-dorsal vein, and attaches to the subadjacent pia. In cases where the middorsal vein is tortuous, the midline dorsal septum is tortuous as well, following the vein in its contours. This midline dorsal septum extends from mid-cervical levels to upper lumbar levels; rostral and caudal to these levels the septum becomes progressively more fenestrated until it is no longer recognizable.[14]

The *dorsolateral septae* are paired attachments of arachnoid which extend from the dorsal root entry zone, envelop the dorsal rootlets and then follow the rootlets laterally. This attachment continues into the root sleeve, where it may distinguish the dorsal rootlets from the ventral rootlets, the latter having no arachnoid covering. The dorsolateral septae are most obvious at thoracic and low cervical levels.[14]

Midway between the dorsal root entry zone and the ventral roots exists a lateral condensation of pia mater referred to as the *dentate* or *denticulate ligament* (*dentate* meaning "sawlike" in Greek). The pial cells of the dentate ligament surround thick collagen bundles. These bundles blend with the subpial collagen surrounding the spinal cord medially while laterally, the dentate attaches to the collagenous dura.[15] The dentate ligaments occur at regular intervals and generally extend rostrally from the entry of the vertebral artery into the subarachnoid space to the caudal T12/L1 area.[14]

The pial covering of the anterior spinal artery forms an irregular longitudinal band referred to as the *linea spendens*. This condensation of pia mater does not attach to the arachnoid.[13,14] The conus medullaris gives rise to a thin ligamentous extension of pia covered by arachnoid cells. This extension is referred to as the *filum terminale internum* (or simply *filum terminale*). A segment of the filum terminale attaches and passes through the caudal-most segment of dura, which in turn is attached to the coccyx; after passing through the dura it is referred to as the *filum terminale externum*.[11,1,5]

2.2 The fine structure of the arachnoid membrane

Ultramicroscopic examination of the arachnoid has revealed two components making up this layer: an outer layer, often referred to as the *arachnoid barrier cell layer*; and an inner layer, often referred to as the *arachnoid trabeculae* (Fig. 1).

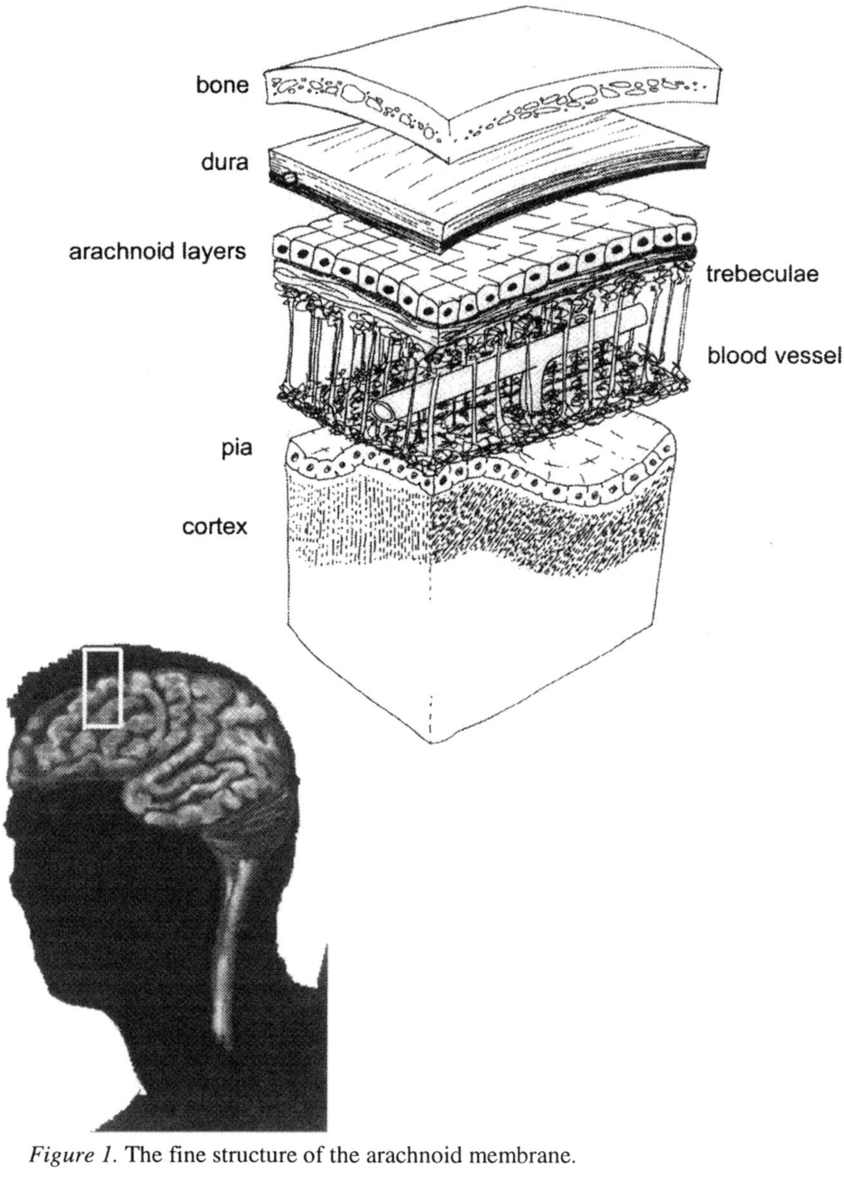

Figure 1. The fine structure of the arachnoid membrane.

The arachnoid barrier cell layer is a layer of two to three tiers of flattened cells. These cells have a large, oval- to spindle-shaped nucleus, multiple cytoplasmic processes, scant mitochondria, small rough endoplasmic reticulum and a poorly developed Gogli apparatus.[5,16,17] These cells are located under the dural border cell layer of the dura mater. A basement membrane underlies the arachnoid barrier cell layer and separates this layer from the underlying subarachnoid space.[5]

The presence of junctional complexes is an important characteristic of the arachnoid barrier cell layer. Numerous zonulae occludens (tight junctions), zonulae adherens, and macula adherens (desmosomes) are found interconnecting cells of this layer. These connections function as the meningeal barrier, which excludes proteins and other large molecules from diffusing from the blood to the CSF in the subarachnoid space.[5,18,17] The function of this barrier may be demonstrated by the intravascular introduction of dyes: the dye will stain the dura but not the underlying meningeal layers, the CSF, or the brain parenchyma.[17]

Occasional intercellular connections (*viz.* desmosomes) also exist between the cells of the arachnoid barrier cell layer in the cranium and the overlying dura. In contrast, intercellular connections between the cells of the dural layers are infrequent. The lack of these intercellular junctions may explain why extravasated blood collects then not in a "potential" subdural space as implied by many textbooks, but in reality, in an *intradural* location (*i.e.* between fine layers of the dura).[5] A final interconnection of note exists between the cells of the arachnoid barrier cell layer and the underlying arachnoid trabecular cells. The trabecular cells penetrate the basement membrane to attach to the arachnoid barrier cell via desmosomes.[5] The *subarachnoid trabeculae* cells are found below the arachnoid barrier cell layer traversing the subarachnoid space as thin, web-like chordae. The arachnoid trabeculae cells are more loosely arranged and more flat in appearance than the arachnoid barrier cells. The cells of the trabecular layer also have smaller nuclei, abundant mitochondria, and well-developed Golgi apparatuses and rough endoplasmic reticulum[16]. Extracellular collagen fibrils are found outside of the cells in this layer.[17]

As mentioned previously, tight junctions are often present in the intercellular connection between cells of the arachnoid barrier and trabecular layers.[5,18]. Gap junctions often connect cells within the arachnoid trabecular layer. The extensive gap junctions allow the arachnoid cells to function together to allow the passage of small molecules from cell to cell.[18]

2.3 The fine structure of the pia mater

The cells of the pia mater are modified fibroblasts similar to the cells of the arachnoid membrane. Their morphology is often undistinguishable from that of the arachnoid cells.[18,19] The pial layer varies in thickness from one to three cells thick.[17] In the cauda equina the pia may be fenestrated[20] leaving the basement membrane of the underlying glial limitans of the parenchyma exposed to the subarachnoid space.[18]

Two layers of the spinal pia were distinguished by Key and Retzius (1875); this distinction has only rarely been referred to by subsequent authors. The outer component has been called the *epipial*[6] or *intermediate leptomeningeal layer*[15] which is a vascular layer present only in the spinal cord. It covers the collagenous core of the denticulate ligament laterally and composes the *linea splendens* anteriorly.[6] The *intimal layer* of pia is an avascular layer found in both the spinal cord (as the inner component) and the brain. In contrast to the overlying epipial layer, it is adherent to the brain and spinal cord throughout all its contours. Blood vessels pierce the intimal pia as they pass into the brain or spinal cord.[15,6] It has been proposed that the vascular epipial layer represents the contribution of mesenchyme to the pia while the avascular intimal layer represents the contribution of the neural crest.[6]

A *subpial space* of variable thickness exists between the pia and the basement membrane of the glial limitans (outer glial layer of the brain and spinal cord). This space contains collagen fibrils.[19] Pial cells are often joined to arachnoid trabecular cells with desmosomes.[5]

2.4 Blood vessels in the subarachnoid space

Blood vessels in the subarachnoid space travel along the outer surface of this space, often suspended from the overlying trabecular layer by chordae composed of arachnoid trabecula cells.[20] It had been previously thought that the pia mater follows the arteries and arterioles for some short distance as they descend into the brain parenchyma. The perivascular space between the descending vessel and the pia, often referred to as the Virchow-Robin space, was thought to communicate with the subarachnoid space. Scanning electron microscopy, however, has revealed that the pia actually surrounds the vessel as it travels through the subarachnoid space but does not accompany the vessel as it descends into the brain parenchyma. Instead, the pia surrounding the vessel spreads out over the pia which is covering the surface of the brain, effectively occluding the perivascular space from the subarachnoid space[20] (Fig. 2). Thus the Virchow-Robin space communicates with the brain extracellular space rather than the subarachnoid space.

A layer of smooth muscle and extracellular matrix separates the pia from the endothelial cells.[18] Similar to the arachnoid cells of the barrier layer, the endothelial cells are interconnected by tight junctions.[17]

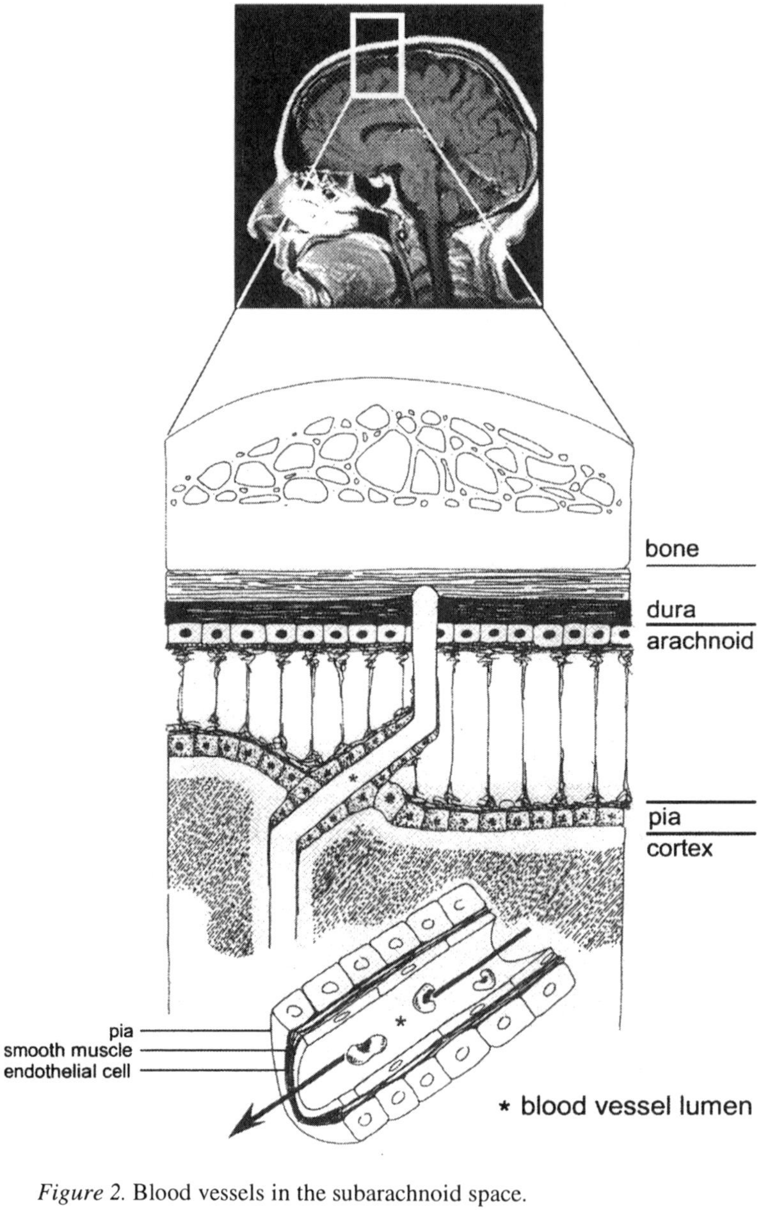

Figure 2. Blood vessels in the subarachnoid space.

2.5 Ependyma

Ependymal cells are found as a monolayer which lines the third and fourth ventricles and the central canal of the spinal cord. Their cell morphology varies, ranging from squamous to cuboid to columnar. Another characteristic is their many cilia. These cilia are associated with a basal body and microtubules with the "9+2" arrangement typical of cilia elsewhere. The nucleus of the cell is oval and regular with an eccentric nucleolus. Organelles such as Golgi and mitochondria are often found in the apical portion of the cell. Ependymal cells are interconnected with fascia adherentes (extensive forms of zonulae adherentes) and gap junctions [[19]].

The primary function of the ependyma may be movement of the CSF caused by beating of the cilia. These cells may also be responsible for trapping foreign cells or microorganisms, and in regenerating ependymal cells. Ependymal cells in the third ventricle may be involved in signaling or transporting molecules to the adenohypophysis.[18]

2.6 Tanycytes and macrophages

Tanycytes are found in clusters in the walls of the third ventricle and cerebral aqueduct, in the floor of the fourth ventricle, and in the cervical spinal canal. Clusters of tanycytes are often associated with circumventricular organs, namely the median eminence, the area postrema, the subcommissural organ, and the pineal gland.[18]

In contrast to the ependymal cells, tanycytes have many microvilli and few cilia. Their nuclei are denser and more elongated than those of the ependymal cells. These cells have three portions: 1) a somatic portion, 2) a neck portion, and 3) a tail portion. The somatic portion is the segment of the cell which rests in the ependymal layer; this section has many lateral cytoplasmic processes. The neck is the portion of the cell which extends into the periventricular neuropil to contact blood vessels. The tail portion features processes with end-feet which course through the hypothalamus to contact fenestrated blood vessels or pial surfaces.[21] The connection that the tanycyte makes between the ventricle and the capillary has led some to conjecture that the tanycyte functions in the transport of hypophysiotropic hormones. However the research supporting this may be inconclusive.

Fixed macrophages are also present in the arachnoid border layer – these cells are sometimes referred to as Kolmer or epiplexus cells when associated with the choroid plexus. They contain many membrane-bound inclusions and variable vacuoles; they lack cytoplasmic processes.[18]

2.7 Choroid plexus

The term *choroid plexus* is most commonly used to refer to the ependymal-derived epithelium which lines the roof of the third and fourth ventricles and the lateral walls of the lateral ventricles. Originally, however, the term choroid plexus referred only to the vasculature underlying this epithelium, while the term *tela choroidea* was used to refer to the choroid plexus vasculature and the overlying epithelium together.[18] Development of the choroid plexus begins as pia. Blood vessels invade the wall of the ventricles, creating folds covered by pseudostratified columnar epithelium. These folds lobulate and eventually the cells become cuboidal-to-squamous in morphology.

The cells feature pale, round central nuclei and apical mitochondria. The luminal surface is lined with both irregular, tightly-packed microvilli and irregular cilia with a "9+2" arrangement of microfilaments. Choroid epithelial cells are joined together with "leaky" tight junctions similar to those found in the gallbladder. Underneath the superficial monolayer of choroidal cells, occasional immature cells can be found. These cells have been shown to take up tritiated thymidine. In primates, renewal of the entire monolayer of choroid has been estimated to occur every one to three years.[19]

The underlying vasculature of the choroid plexus is notable for its fenestrated, thin-walled, relatively large-diameter capillaries. The arterial supply to the choroid plexus of the lateral ventricles is supplied via the anterior and posterior choroidal arteries; the anterior is a segment directly derived from the internal carotid while the posterior is a branch of the posterior cerebral artery. The choroid plexus of the third ventricle is supplied by choroidal branches of the posterior cerebral artery, while the choroid plexus of the fourth ventricle is supplied by the posterior inferior cerebellar artery with possible supplementation from the anterior inferior cerebellar artery and the internal auditory artery. The thalamostriate and internal cerebral veins drain the majority of the blood from the choroid plexus of the lateral and third ventricles; most of the blood from the choroid plexus of the fourth ventricle is drained by the basal vein of Rosenthal.[22] The choroid plexus has a rich autonomic innervation supplied by the cervical sympathetic chain and the vagus.[21]

2.8 Arachnoid villi and granulations

Arachnoid granulations were first illustrated by Vesalius who observed their imprint on the inner surface of the skull. Pacchioni described the structures, but mistakenly thought that they were lymph nodes which irrigated the meninges. Faivre is accredited with correctly proposing that the granulations serve to drain CSF.[2]

These leptomeningeal structures are often thought of as one-way valves from the CSF compartment to the venous compartment. They are commonly called *arachnoid villi* when microscopic or *arachnoid granulations* when macroscopic. The name *Pacchionian granulation* has been used to refer to large, elaborate arachnoid granulations in horses and in man.[23]

Harvey Cushing, in his 1901 Mütter lecture, proposed that the arachnoid villi functioned as one-way valves similar to the valves in the lymphatic system (*i.e.* an "open" system). At the same time, L.H. Weed, a researcher in the Hunterian labs, found no structures which resembled valves upon light microscopic examination of the villi. He found only an intact membrane covering the villi, and proposed that transcellular transportation occurred via pinocytosis (*i.e.* a "closed" system).[24]

The advent of electron microscopy led to re-examination of the functional anatomy of the arachnoid villi and helped establish the fact that micropinocytosis does indeed contribute to the unidirectional flow of CSF.[25,26] The presence of unidirectional valves has been found in monkeys and there is some evidence that widened intercellular gaps contribute to the unidirectional flow of CSF in humans as well.[27] However, the question of whether the system is "open" or "closed" (or a combination) remains to be answered definitively.

2.9 The cerebral spinal fluid space

The CSF circulates between the ventricles within the brain and a series of cisterns and spaces outside the brain and spinal cord. While the ventricles are lined with ependymal cells, the cisterns and spaces outside the brain are lined with arachnoid and pial cells.

The paired lateral ventricles are often divided into five sections. From anterior to posterior these sections are: 1) the anterior (frontal) horn, 2) the body, 3) the atrium (trigone), 4) the posterior (occipital) horn, and 5) the inferior (temporal) horn. As stated above, the medial walls of the lateral ventricles are lined with choroid plexus. Interestingly, while the central nervous system contains approximately 130 mL of CSF, only some 18 mL are contained in the lateral ventricles.

The third ventricle, only a few milliliters in volume, is a midline cavity whose roof is lined with choroid plexus. The interthalamic adhesion is a solid structure which traverses the cavity. Numerous recesses are present in the third ventricle. Among them are the optic, infundibular, pineal, and suprapineal recess.[1,11]

The fourth ventricle is located between the cerebellum, the pons, and the medulla. It is shaped like a rhomboid with paired lateral recesses found at its widest portion. The inferior half of the roof of the fourth ventricle, referred to as the inferior medullary velum, is lined with choroid plexus[11,1]

A number of CSF cisterns in the subarachnoid space have been described.[1,11,12]

3. PRODUCTION AND COMPOSITION OF THE CEREBROSPINAL FLUID

A major advance in localizing the site of CSF production was made by Dandy in 1919 when he completed a crucial experiment by stenosing both foramina of Monroe and performing a unilateral choroid plexectomy in a single dog. After the observing that the ventricle without choroid plexus collapsed, while the opposite ventricle expanded greatly, it was initially thought that the sole source of CSF was localized to the choroid plexus [[29]]. Currently it is believed that while the choroid plexus is an important site of CSF production, other significant sources exist. They include the ependyma and the brain parenchyma.[21] Indeed, it has been estimated that approximately 30% of CSF is produced by the ependyma.[28]

The CSF is not simply a protein-free dialysate of the plasma, but rather a true secretion requiring energy for its production. The secretion of CSF is dependent upon the active transport of sodium which is performed by a choroid epithelial sodium-potassium activated ATPase. The *in vivo* inhibition of choroid plexus fluid formation by ouabain, an inhibitor of this ATPase, supports the idea that CSF is a secretion. This ATPase and other transport enzymes are responsible for the transport of other ions and micronutrients into the CSF. Small amounts of protein are transported into the CSF mainly by pinocytosis. The fact that the CSF is isosmotic in comparison to the plasma suggests that water freely equilibrates between the two fluid compartments.[21] The composition of CSF compared to that of plasma is presented in Table 2.

Table 2: Normal Composition of Cerebrospinal Fluid and Serum (adapted from[21])

	CSF	Serum (arterial)
Osmolarity (mOsm/L)	295	295
Water content (%)	99	93
Sodium (mEq/L)	138	138
Potassium (mEq/L)	2.8	4.5
Chloride (mEq/L)	119	102
Bicarbonate (mEq/L)	22.0	24.0
Phosphorus (mg/dL)	1.6	4.0
Calcium (mEq/L)	2.1	4.8
Magnesium (mEq/L)	2.3	1.7
Iron (g/dL)	1.5	15.0
Urea (mmol/dL)	4.7	5.4
Creatinine (mg/dL)	1.2	1.8
Uric acid (mg/dL)	0.25	5.50
CO_2 tension (mmHg)	47.0	41.0
pH	7.33	7.41
Oxygen (mmHg)	43.0	104.0
Glucose (mg/dL)	60.0	90.0
Lactate (mEq/L)	1.6	1.0
Pyruvate (mEq/L)	0.08	0.11
Lactate:pyruvate ratio	26.0	17.6
Proteins (gm/dL)	0.035	7.0

3.1 Pulsatile movement and circulation of the CSF

Until Cushing's paper The Third Circulation in 1925, most had ascribed to the idea that CSF moved with an "ebb and flow" movement, an idea begun by Magendie 100 years before.[28] Modern radiological techniques confirmed the notion that the CSF does indeed circulate.[29,30,31] CSF formed in the lateral ventricles flows into the third ventricle via the paired interventricular foramina of Monroe. The fluid then flows from the third ventricle to the fourth ventricle via the cerebral aqueduct (Aqueduct of Sylvius) then out of the fourth ventricle and into the cisterna magna via the paired lateral apertures (foramina of Luschka) and the unpaired median aperture (the foramen of Magendie).[1]

Many different routes are possible once the CSF fluid has reached the cisterna magna. The fluid may travel: (1) superiorly toward the cerebellar hemispheres to the ambient cistern; (2) anterosuperiorly toward the interpeduncular and interchiasmatic cisterns; (2) anteriorly toward the premedullary, prepontine, and cerebellopontine cisterns; or (4) inferiorly toward the spinal subarachnoid space. CSF in the spinal subarachnoid space posterior to the spinal cord and dentate ligaments is directed in the caudal direction. The fluid may reach as far caudal as the lumbar thecal sac before it circulates anteriorly to the ventral spinal subarachnoid space. The overall direction of fluid ventral to the spinal cord is in the cephalad direction; therefore, returning the CSF to the basilar cisterns.[28]

Several mechanisms have been proposed to account for the circulation of the CSF. Perhaps the smallest contribution is from the outpouring of new CSF and the ciliary beating of the ventricular ependyma. The pressure gradient across the arachnoid villi also contributes to the bulk flow of CSF via the creation of a pressure gradient. The mean CSF pressure in the brain is 150 mm saline while the pressure in the superior sagittal sinus is 90 mm saline.[28] The flow of CSF is also propagated by the cardiac cycle. The pulsation of the arterial system transmits pulsations to the brain parenchyma, the choroid plexus, and the large arteries at the skull base.[31] The volumetric displacement of the CSF increases with low diastolic pressure and low systolic pressure.

The amplitude of the CSF pulsations is also affected by: 1) the respiratory cycle, 2) the resistance to outflow created by the arachnoid villi, 3) the mean intracranial pressure, and 4) the compliance of the cranial and spinal cord cavities.[22,31] Pulsations of 10-30 mm H_2O and 20-30 mm H_2O in amplitude are seen at particular points in the respiratory and cardiac cycles, respectively, with isovolumetric measurements in the lumbar CSF.[22] The amplitude of pulsations decreases as one proceeds caudally along the neuraxis; i.e., the amplitude of pulsations in the cisterna magna is 50 mm H_2O while that of the lumbar fluid is 30 mm H_2O.[21]

The pulsation of the third ventricle was initially thought to represent a "CSF pump", i.e., that the expansion of the brain parenchyma during systole was thought to compress the third ventricle, forcing CSF out via through the cerebral aqueduct with each heart beat. However, more recent radiographic studies in humans have shown that pulsations *throughout* the neuraxis lead to the "pumping" of CSF and that various areas of the brain and spinal cord provide varying contributions to the pumping activity. Duboulay *et al* showed that an average of 0.1 mL CSF was displaced from the third ventricle during each systole; in comparison to 1.0 mL in the basal cisterns and 0.64 mL in the cisterna magna.[29]

3.2 CSF absorption

The majority of the CSF produced appears to be absorbed across the arachnoid villi and into the venous circulation. Other routes of absorption exist, however, including the ependyma, the leptomeninges, and the lymphatics of the spine.[28] The driving forces for absorption of CSF have been attributed to the gradients in both hydrostatic and colloid osmotic pressures, which exist between the protein-free CSF in the arachnoid villi and the venous spaces. However, if the absorption of CSF does indeed occur across an intact membrane (*i.e.* a "closed" system -- see above) the contribution of colloid osmotic pressure in the net flow of CSF across the villi would be less likely.[28]

3.3 CSF function

As one of its functions, the CSF does act to support and cushion elements of the central nervous system (CNS). Considering the difference in specific gravity between the brain and the cerebrospinal fluid (1.040 from the brain vs. 1.007 for the CSF), the CSF acts to lessen the apparent weight of the brain to approximately 4% of its mass.[11]

Yet consistent with the complex mechanisms for its circulation, formation and absorption, the function of CSF appears to be more complex than simply that of acting as a "cushion" to protect the brain. The CSF appears have a function at least partially analogous to that of the lymphatics in other organs -- namely, removing fat-soluble and toxic substances from the brain's extracellular fluid (ECF). Many fat-insoluble molecules are also removed from the brain ECF by the circulation of the CSF including urea, albumin, homovanillic acid, and norepinephrine.[28]

The "internal milieu" of the brain (i.e. the brain's ECF) may be regulated to a large part by the CSF. This regulation occurs by exclusion of large and polar molecules from the CSF and also by modification of the CSF by capillary-glial complexes, epithelia, and neurons themselves.[21] Finally, the CSF may function as a mechanism of intracerebral transport for biogenic amines which initiate the secretion of pituitary hormone release factors. Tanyctes appear to have a role in this function.[28]

References

1. Nolte J. The Human Brain: An introduction to Its functional anatomy. St. Louis: Mosby Year Book, 1993; 33-47.
2. Bakay L. Discovery of the arachnoid membrane. Surg Neurol 1991; 36:63-68.
3. Sanan A, van Loveren HR. The arachnoid and the Myth of Arachne. Neurosurgery 1999; 45:152.
4. Key A, Retzius G. Studien in der anatomie des nervensystems. Samson & Wallin, Stockholm, 1876.
5. Haines DE, Frederickson RG. The Meninges. In: Al-Mefty O. Meningiomas. New York, Raven Press, 1991, pp 9-25.
6. Millen JW, Woollam HM. On the nature of the pia mater. Brain 1961; 84:514-520.
7. Senesing EC. The early development of the meninges of the spinal cord in human embryos. *Carngie Contributions to Embryology.* Carnegie Institution of Washington 1951;34:147-164.
8. Pansky B. Review of Medical Embryology. New York, MacMillian Publishing Company, Inc., 1982.
9. McLone DG, Bondareff W. Developmental morphology of the subarachnoid space and contiguous structures in the mouse. Am J Anat 1975; 142: 273-294.
10. Moore KL, Persaud TVN. The Developing Human. Philadelphia: W.B. Saunders Co., 1993, pp 385-422.
11. Burt AM. Textbook of Neuroanatomy. Philadelphia:W.B.Saunders Co, 1993.
12. Yasargil MG, Kasdaglis K, Jain KK, Weber HP. Anatomical observations of the subarachnoid cisterns of the brain during surgery. J Neurosurg 1976; 44:298-302.
13. Moore KL. Clinically Oriented Anatomy. Baltimore, Williams & Wilkins, 1992, pp 366-8.
14. Nauta HJW, Dolan E, Yasargil MG. Microsurgical anatomy of spinal subarachnoid space. Surg Neurol 1983; 19:431-7.
15. Nicholas DS, Weller RO. The fine anatomy of the human spinal meninges. J Neurosurg 1988; 69:276-282.
16. Oba Y, Nakanishi I. Ultrastructure of the mouse leptomeninx. J Comp Neur 1984; 225: 448-457.
17. Nabeshima S, Reese TS, Landis DMD, Brightman MW. Junctions in the meninges and marginal glia. J Comp Neur 1975; 164: 127-134.
18. Peters A, Palay SL, Webster H. The Fine Structure of the Nervous System. New York: Oxford University Press, 1991.
19. Cloyd MW, Low FN. Scanning electron microscopy of the subarachnoid space in the dog. J Comp Neurol 1974; 153:325-368.
20. Hutchings M, Weller RO. Anatomical relationships of the pia mater to cerebral blood vessels in man. J Neurosurg 1985; 65:316-325.
21. Fishman RA. Cerebrospinal Fluid in Diseases of the Nervous System. Philadelphia:W.B.Saunders Co, 1992.
22. Fujii K, Lentely C, Rhoton AL Jr. Microsurgical anatomy of the choroid arteries: Lateral and third ventricles. J Neurosurg 1980; 52:165-188.
23. Wolpow ER, Schaumburg HH. Structure of the human arachnoid granulation. J Neurosurg 1972; 37:724-727.
24. Welch K, Friedman V. The cerebrospinal fluid valves. Brain 1960; 83:454-469.
25. Alksne JF, Lovings ET. Functional ultrastructure of the arachnoid villus. Arch Neurol 1972; 27:371-377.
26. Tripathi BS, Tripathi RC. Vacuolar transcellular channels as a drainage pathway for cerebrospinal fluid. J Physiol 1974; 239:195-206.
27. Yamashima T. Functional ultrastructure of cerebrospinal fluid drainage Channels in Human Arachnoid Villi. Neurosurgery 1988; 22: 633-641.

28. Milhorat TH. The third circulation revisited. J Neurosurg 1975; 42:628-645.
29. DuBoulay G, O'Connel J, Currie J, Bostch T, Verity P. Further investigation on the pulsatile movements in the cerebrospinal fluid pathway. Acta Radiol 1972; 13:496-523.
30. Stoodley MA, Brown SA, Brown CJ, Jones NR. Arterial pulsation-dependent perivascular cerebrospinal fluid flow into the central canal in sheep spinal cord. J Neurosurg 1997; 86:686-693.
31. Ohara S, Nagain H, Matsumoto T, Banno T. MR imaging of the CSF pulsatory flow and its relation to intracranial pressure. J Neurosurg 1988; 69:675-682.

Chapter 2

LEPTOMENINGEAL NEOPLASIA: EPIDEMIOLOGY, CLINICAL PRESENTATION, CSF ANALYSIS AND DIAGNOSTIC IMAGING

Roelien H. Enting, M.D.
University Hospital Groningen, The Netherlands

Abstract: The incidence of leptomeningeal metastasis over the past several decades has increased among solid tumor patients and decerased in patients with hematologic malignancies. Improvements in systemic therapies are likely responsible for both changes; solid tumor patients are living longer and, threfore, are at higher risk to develop leptomeningeal tumors while patients with hematologic malignancy have benefitted from more aggressive central nervous system prophylaxis. Regardless, both types of patients present with symptoms referrable to multiple levels of the central nervous system and a careful dignostic approach incorporating cerebrospinal fluid studies and appropriate neuroimaging is critical.

Key words: Leptomeningeal metastases; clinical features; diagnosis; CSF cytology; neuroimaging

1. INTRODUCTION

Historically, leptomeningeal metastases (LM) were often diagnosed at autopsy; however, autopsy results vary widely depending on institution and whether or not the spinal cord was examined.[1] Among 2375 autopsies of patients with cancer, leptomeningeal metastases occurred in 8%, and in 3% tumor was limited to the leptomeninges. The highest rates of LM without other central nervous system (CNS) metastases were seen in acute lymphocytic leukemia, non-Hodgkin's lymphoma, breast cancer, melanoma, acute myelogenous leukemia, lung, and gastrointestinal cancer (listed in decreasing order of frequency).[1] Cancer patients with neurological signs at multiple levels of the neuraxis, or with neurological symptoms attributable to the leptomeningeal space, e.g., an isolated cranial neuropathy, should be suspected to have leptomeningeal metastases.[2,3,4] Since these symptoms might also be explained by epidural, dural or parenchymatous metastases, or non-cancer related causes, the work-up should begin with neuroimaging.[3] The first choice is a magnetic resonance image (MRI); the combination of non-enhanced FLAIR and contrast-enhanced T1-weighted image has proved to be optimal.[5,6] The next step should be a lumbar puncture in order to examine the cerebrospinal fluid for pathologic cells. The sensitivity of cytology is far from optimal, but the specificity is estimated to be greater than 95%.[7,8,9] Patients may be diagnosed with LM when one of the following criteria is met: 1) a positive cerebrospinal fluid cytology; 2) a positive LM biopsy, 3) a positive MRI in a patient with a clinical syndrome compatible with the diagnosis, or 4) abnormal CSF biochemical markers consistent with LM.[10] Since different definitions of LM have been used in the literature, it may be difficult to evaluate the sensitivity and specificity of the various procedures used to diagnose LM.

2. STAGING AND CLASSIFICATION

LM may arise at any time during the course of cancer. In up to 30% of patients, LM is the first presentation of cancer.[7,11-14] However, the majority of patients will have widespread disease when LM is diagnosed.[14-17] In a report from a cytopathology laboratory, LM was the initial presentation of cancer in 11% of 200 specimens in which malignant cells were identified. Among patients with LM as their first presentation, the distribution of the underlying neoplasms was as follows; 2% of patients with leukemia or lymphoma, 18% of patients with lung cancer, 8% of patients with melanoma, 71% of patients with unknown primary, and 50% of patients with primary brain tumors. No patient with breast cancer presented with LM.[7] A small subset of patients with a known history of cancer develop LM as an isolated site of recurrence without evidence of simultaneous systemic relapse.[1,10,14,18-21] LM was seen in conjunction with other CNS metastases (brain parenchymal, dural or epidural), in-one third of patients in a clinical series, and two-thirds of patients in an autopsy study.[1,3]

Classifications have been developed for the extent of LM in leukemia, lymphoma, and medulloblastoma, but different research groups use different criteria.[22-28] In the pediatric literature, controversy exists regarding the significance of blasts detected in CSF without pleocytosis. Therefore, CNS status in leukemic patients is usually categorized as one of the following; CNS-1, nontraumatic puncture without leukemic blasts after cytocentrifugation; CNS-2, nontraumatic puncture, ≤5 WBC/μL with identifiable blasts; CNS-3, nontraumatic puncture, >5 WBC/μL with identifiable blasts; TLP+, traumatic puncture with blasts; TLP-, traumatic puncture without blasts.[22,23] The threshold to diagnose CNS involvement in acute myelogenous leukemia (AML) also differs between research groups. To some, any blast cells in the CSF is sufficient for the diagnosis, whereas others use a threshold of 5 or 10 WBC/μl. Furthermore, some consider the presence of cranial neuropathy as sufficient for the diagnosis of LM.[24] The criteria for LM in non-Hodgkin's lymphoma is blasts in the CSF, or the presence of a cranial neuropathy.[25,27-29] The criteria for LM in medulloblastoma are shown in Table 1.

Table1. Chang classification of tumor and metastasis stage for medulloblastoma

M stage	
M0	No gross subarachnoid or hematogenous metastasis
M1	Microscopic tumor cells found in CSF
M2	Gross nodular seeding in cerebellum, cerebral subarachnoid space, or in third or fourth ventricle
M3	Gross nodular seeding in spinal subarachnoid space
M4	Extraneuraxial metastasis

3. INCIDENCE

The observed incidence of LM from solid tumors appears to be increasing for a variety of reasons. First, cytologic methods of diagnosis have improved. Second, as patients with cancer continue to live longer, this complication has more time to develop. Third, improvements in imaging may contribute to the increasing incidence.[30] On the other hand, intrathecal prophylaxis has caused LM to become less common in patients with leukemia and non-Hodgkin's lymphoma.[1,3] Therefore, the data concerning the incidence of LM will be considered separately for solid tumors, hematological malignancies, or primary CNS tumors.

4. SOLID TUMORS

In patients autopsied between 1970-1976 at Memorial Sloan-Kettering Cancer Center, LM was seen as the sole intracranial metastasis in 5% of patients with melanoma, 3% of patients with breast cancer, 1% of patients with lung cancer, gastrointestinal cancer or sarcoma.[31,32] Current epidemiologic studies suggest that 3-8% of solid tumor patients will develop LM during the course of their illness.[33-35] In particular, patients with breast cancer, melanoma and small cell lung cancer are at high risk of LM dissemination. In a series of 122 patients with advanced melanoma, 11% of patients had clinical signs of LM, and in a subset of patients who underwent autopsy, 52% had meningeal infiltration often with concomitant brain metastases.[32] LM was documented in 11% of 526 patients with small cell lung cancer treated at the National Cancer Institute between 1969 and 1980; the probability of developing LM increased with survival from 0.5% at diagnosis to 25% at three years. LM was seen in 26% of autopsies.[14]

5. HEMATOLOGICAL MALIGNANCIES

Approximately 10-30% of patients with acute leukemia will have LM dissemination at diagnosis; children, particularly those younger than two years and patients with AML are at highest risk.[36-39] However, aggressive combined modality treatment with disease-specific CNS prophylaxis has dramatically decreased the risk of LM relapse to less than 5%.[22] A notable exception is acute promyelocytic leukemia where the rate of LM relapse has increased since the incorporation of all trans-retinoic acid in routine maintenance therapy.[40,41] LM dissemination is rarely seen in patients with CLL, CML or multiple myeloma.[42,43,44]

The risk of LM ranges between 5% and 30% in all NHL subtypes, with a cumulative risk of LM at four years of 17%. Overall, LM is observed in <3% of indolent lymphomas, 5% of aggressive lymphomas (diffuse large B-cell and peripheral T-cell lymphomas) and 24% of Burkitt's and lymphoblastic lymphomas.[43,46,47,52,53] The analysis of risk factors for LM in NHL is limited by differences in the definition criteria and retrospective nature of reported studies. Nevertheless, several variables including advanced disease, increased serum levels of lactate dehydrogenase, certain extranodal sites of disease, and highly aggressive lymphoma histologies have been associated with an increased risk for CNS recurrence in NHL.

Nearly 5% of patients with large B-cell lymphoma develop LM, with an actuarial risk at one year after diagnosis of 4.5%. This risk can be reduced to <2% if patients are treated with chemotherapy that includes intrathecal and systemic HD-MTX.[48,49,50] In 20% of cases, LM recurrence is concurrent with early systemic progression but, in 30% of cases, it precedes systemic progression by up to six months and isolated LM recurrence has been observed in 5% of patients with aggressive lymphomas treated without intrathecal chemotherapy. While testicular lymphoma has been noted to have a high rate of CNS relapse, most patients have isolated parenchymal brain relapse or parenchymal brain relapse with LM.[51]

6. PRIMARY CENTRAL NERVOUS SYSTEM TUMORS

Leptomeningeal dissemination of primary CNS tumors is relatively rare, but is clinically relevant for patients with medulloblastoma, primary CNS lymphomas and germ cell tumors. Twenty-five (50%) of patients with medulloblastoma will have evidence of LM dissemination at diagnosis; this is a critical factor in determining appropriate therapy and overall prognosis.[57,58,59] Approximately 25-30% of patients with primary central nervous system lymphoma (PCNSL) have LM dissemination at diagnosis. This should suggest the need for IT therapy and may portend a poor outcome.[54] Fewer than 10% of other primary CNS tumors, such as glioma[56] and ependymoma[55], may seed the CSF space resulting in dropped metastases and discontiguous neurologic signs or symptoms. Of note, neuroimaging may be more sensitive than CSF cytology in the detection of dropped metastases from glioma or ependymoma.[56]

7. CLINICAL FEATURES

Patients typically present with multi-focal symptoms and signs related to different levels of the neuraxis (Table 2).[1,3,60-63] Frequent cerebral signs or symptoms include headache, change in mental status, nausea and vomiting, or seizures. Common spinal complaints, e.g. weakness, paresthesias in one or more extremities, back pain, radicular pain, and bladder or bowel dysfunction; associated findings include asymmetries of deep tendon reflexes, nuchal rigidity or pain on straight leg raising. The most common cranial nerve complaints are diplopia, facial numbness, hearing loss, and loss of visual acuity.[(3)]

Table 2. A summary of symptoms and / or signs of LM (n=799)

Reference	*2*	*19*	*15*	*14*	*64*	*3*	*49*	*65*	*16*	*66*	*12*	*33*	*67*	*10*	*11*	*34*
N	*50*	*25*	*33*	*60*	*105*	*90*	*38*	*44*	*90*	*63*	*34*	*35*	*126*	*32*	*45*	*19*
Cancer type	*S, H*	*S*	*S*	*S*	*H*	*S*	*H*	*S, H*	*H*	*S,H*	*S*	*S*	*S*	*S*	*S, H*	*S*
	%	*%*	*%*	*%*	*%*	*%*	*%*	*%*	*%*	*%*	*%*	*%*	*%*	*%*	*%*	*%*
Ccerebral	*40*	*64*	*ns*	*68*	*ns*	*50*	*ns*	*ns*	*ns*	ns	*ns*	*ns*	ns	*ns*	*36*	*ns*
Headache	38	52	39	10	31	33	29	48	23	32	65	ns	51	32	ns	79
Altered mental status	24	48	54	60	29	17	21	23	42	63	15	6	26	3	ns	53
Dizziness	14	24	ns	2	ns	2	ns	7	ns	ns	ns	ns	ns	ns	ns	ns
Nausea or vomiting	12	32	12	3	16	11	18	16	ns	ns	21	ns	34	ns	ns	ns
Seizures	8	8	3	0	3	6	8	9	3	14	12	9	18	ns	ns	26
Ataxic gait	10	ns	36	3	5	13	ns	25	ns	22	ns	9	20	16	ns	16
	78	*52*	*ns*	*18*	*50*	*56*	*60*	*ns*	*36*	*49*	*ns*	*31*	*ns*	*28*	*44*	*ns*
Cranial nerves																
III, IV, VI	46	44	39	7	26	20	47	ns	19	ns	41	29	29	22	ns	33
VII	42	24	30	10	14	17	21	ns	18	ns	26	ns	10	6	ns	7
VIII	30	24	3	2	5	10	ns	ns	1	ns	59	ns	7	ns	ns	13
II	14	ns	ns	3	4	6	ns	ns	1	ns	44	ns	19	ns	ns	0
V	12	ns	18	2	8	6	ns	ns	8	ns	6	ns	6	ns	ns	0
XII	8	ns	ns	3	ns	6	ns	ns	4	ns	15	ns	5	ns	ns	0
	40	*28*	*ns*	*67*	*ns*	*82*	*ns*	*ns*	*44*	*ns*	*ns*	*ns*	*ns*	*25*	*47*	*ns*
Spinal																
Lower motor weakness	22	28	34	57	22	38	29	36	ns	38	9	9	34	Ns	ns	37
Paresthesias	10	ns	ns	10	ns	34	8	20	ns	ns	41	ns	ns	ns	ns	ns
Radicular pain	12	ns	ns	ns	ns	21	ns	ns	ns	ns	9	ns	ns	ns	ns	ns
Back / neck Pain	18	16	ns	18	20	26	2	32	ns	76	47	ns	37	ns	ns	ns
Bowel / bladder dysfunction	2	20	ns	20	7	13	ns	4	ns	19	9	ns	ns	ns	ns	16

8. CSF ANALYSIS

CSF analysis is the gold standard for the diagnosis of LM. Most authors agree that in the absence of large posterior fossa lesions, lesions completely obstructing the flow of CSF, or lesions causing severe mass effect and evidence of herniation, no contraindication exists to performing a lumbar puncture.[61] The CSF is abnormal in nearly all patients, but many abnormalities are non-specific (Table 3). [2,3,12,15,19,49,65-67]

Table 3. CSF findings initial lumbar puncture (n=491)

Reference	2	15	3	49	19	65	66	12	67
Cancer type	S, H	S	S	H	S	S, H	S, H	S	S
N =	47	28	90	34	25	44	63	34	126
Elevated pressure	57%	36%	50%	ns	ns	70%	ns	26%	ns
Elevated cells	57%	68%	57%	94%	ns	ns	74%	94%	79%
Elevated protein	74%	86%	81%	85%	68%	80%	61%	85%	86%
Decreased glucose	40%	64%	31%	Ns	44%	55%	47%	38%	56%
Positive cytology	45%	86%	54%	79%	92%	75%	71%	94%	75%
Normal	0%	ns	3%	ns	ns	ns	ns	0%	0%

S, solid cancer; H, hematological malignancies; ns, not stated

CSF biochemical markers including lactate dehydrogenase-5 (LDH-5), carcinoembryonic antigen (CEA), β2-microglobulin, soluble CD27, or β-glucuronidase are non-specific but may be used to support the diagnosis of LM. In contrast, CSF cytology is highly specific; false-positive results are rare and both intra and inter observer variation is minimal.[7,68] The major drawback of CSF cytology is the low sensitivity.[3,8] The initial CSF is positive in 45 to 94% and this rate may increase to more than 80% when the procedure is repeated (Table 4).[2,3,8,10-13,15,16,19-21,33,34,66,67,69-71]

Table 4. CSF pathology in repeated lumbar punctures (% positive findings) (N=874)

Ref.	**Definition of LM**	**Cancer type**	**Initial CSF**	**2 nd CSF**	**3 rd CSF**	**All CSF samples**
15	positive cytology	S	85%	ns	ns	100%
66	positive cytology	S, H	71%	92%	ns	100%
19	positive cytology	S	92%	100%		
76	positive cytology	S	91%	98%	100%	
34	positive cytology	S	89%	100%		
12	positive cytology	S	94%	ns	ns	100%
34	Histologically proven	S	ns	ns	ns	59%
2	Histologically proven	S, H	45%	64%	72%	75%
8	Histologically proven	S, H, P	ns	ns	ns	59%
82	Histologically proven	S, H	63%	78%	88%	88%
33	Histologically proven	S	91%	97%	nd	
67	Histologically proven	S	75%	92%	94%	nd
70	Positive cytology/exclusion	S	59%	71%	79%	90%
16	Histologically proven/exclusion	H	ns	81%	85%	
71	Positive cytology or MRI	S, H	57%	72%	74%	nd
10	Positive cytology or exclusion	S	66%	78%	81%	nd
11	Histologically proven/exclusion	S, H	67%	ns	ns	84%
3	Positive cytology/exclusion	S	54%	84%	86%	87%

S, solid cancer; H, hematological malignancy; P, primary brain tumor; ns, not stated; nd, not done;

Four hypothesized sources of false-negative results were examined in 39 untreated patients prospectively: volume error, site error, handling error, and sampling frequency error. The false-negative rate for 7.0 mL samples was estimated at 10%, and for 10.5 mL samples at 3%. Significantly larger than expected false-negative rates were observed when CSF was obtained from a location remote from the site of clinical or radiological disease (i.e., lumbar fluid in the setting of cranial signs or symptoms, or ventricular fluid in the setting of spinal signs or symptoms). The false-negative error rate after a 48-hour delay in processing was 36%. From this study it was concluded that the initial diagnosis of LM is established most reliably when a volume of 10.5 mL is processed, with CSF obtained near the site of clinical or radiological disease, when processing is not delayed (and therefore not at night, or over the weekend). The question of how many samplings are necessary is a much debated issue, but in general, very high yields are obtained after two samplings, and little additional benefit was gained by subsequent sampling.[9] The shedding of malignant cells into the CSF most likely occurs intermittently; therefore, a single CSF specimen, no matter how large, expeditiously handled, or appropriately obtained from a symptomatic site, may fail to capture malignant cells.[9] It has been found that within 90 minutes, 90% of cells are lysed when CSF is kept at room temperature.[72]

Newer laboratory techniques utilizing monoclonal antibodies, flow cytometry, polymerase chain reaction for clonal immunoglobulin gene rearrangement, fluorescent in situ hybridization (FISH) for aberrant numbers of chromosome copies, and immunohistochemical techniques are available for diagnosis, and may be helpful in patients strongly suspected of having LM.[62,73] Flow cytometry allows detection of an abnormal population in samples with little cellularity that otherwise might have been not detected when morphologic examination alone was used. Flow cytometry appears especially useful for the diagnosis of lymphoma or leukemia in CSF which may be difficult because of the presence of normal or reactive lymphocytes, or by scant cells in the sample. The major drawback is that approximately 5% of samples cannot be analyzed because of too few cells.[74] Among 21 samples that revealed lymphomatous involvement of the CSF, 57% were diagnosed by both cytology and flow cytometry, and 43% by flow cytometry alone suggesting an improved sensitivity.[41]

Immunohistochemical analysis of the first sample of CSF using tumor specific monoclonal antibodies showed very few patients where the immunohistochemical analysis was positive when the cytology was negative, but the converse was often observed. Therefore, this technique is not useful as a screening test, but may be helpful when cytology fails in a patient who is strongly suspected of having LM.[75-77] Preliminary reports have suggested that special techniques may increase the yield of immunohistochemistry.[78] Polymerase chain reaction (PCR)-based monitoring allows detection of small numbers of malignant cells not detectable with conventional techniques. PCR may be useful for early detection of CNS relapse in ALL or lymphoma or for negative cytology samples.[79-81] However, sensitivity and specificity of these techniques have not yet been thoroughly studied.

9. DIAGNOSTIC IMAGING

Contrast-enhanced MRI reveals abnormalities in up to 80% of patients with LM, but the specificity of abnormal MRI findings is not optimal.[5,6,71,88-91] Neuroimaging findings are more likely to be abnormal in patients with solid tumors (90-100%) than in those with hematological malignancies (40-55%).[88,89]

MRI findings often yield complimentary CSF cytology and diagnostic information (Table 5). As LP may result in meningeal enhancement, patients suspected of LM should undergo neuroimaging prior to LP. MRI scans that show clear leptomeningeal or subependymal enhancement in either the brain (indicated by enhancement extending into the sulci of the cerebral hemispheres or into the folia of the cerebellum), spinal cord, or cauda equina can be considered diagnostic of LM in the appropriate clinical context. Scans with dural enhancement (focal or diffuse enhancement over the convexity of the brain surface but not extending into sulci), superficial cerebral lesions in close proximity to the subarachnoid space or within sulci, enhancement of cranial nerves, or communicating hydrocephalus should suggest the possibility of LM.[88] Alternatively, the categories of 'positive' and 'suggestive' are taken together.[71] An MRI fluid-attenuated inversion-recovery (FLAIR) image demonstrating abnormally high signal intensity in the cisterns, ventricles, sulci, or any pial surface is also consistent with the diagnosis of LM. A comparison of available MRI found that unenhanced FLAIR images had a sensitivity of 12%, contrast-enhanced FLAIR images had a sensitivity of 41%, and contrast-enhanced T1-weighted images had a sensitivity of 59%; the combined overall sensitivity is 65%.[5,6]

Table 5. MRI vs CSF cytology findings

Study Ref.	% Patients with LM based on CSF, MRI or both	Positive CSF cytology	Positive MRI	Both positive
59	32%	35%	26%	38%
71	77%	19%	26%	55%
89	73%	43%	25%	32%

A gadolinium enhanced MRI is positive in approximately half of patients with LMD. In one series, 57% were positive at multiple levels; the cervical spine was involved in 38%, the thoracic spine in 54% and the lumbar spine in 89%. The enhancement pattern was diffuse in 53%, nodular in 37% and combined in 10%. The MRI was positive in 49% of patients without symptoms suggestive of spinal involvement, and in 84% of patients with spinal signs or symptoms. In the latter group, 42% had MRI abnormalities only at the clinically suspected level, and the remaining patients had abnormalities at additional levels as well. The high rate of involvement of the lower spinal column may justify an enhanced-only MRI study of the lumbar spine as an efficient screen for LM in the high risk patient with negative cytology and no localized findings.[92]

In summary, cancer patients with LM dissemination present with signs or symptoms that may be attributed to multiple levels of the neuraxis. A contrast-enhanced MRI of the symptomatic level is the first step to exclude parenchymatous, dural, skull base or epidural metastases and to look for radiographic evidence of LM. A contrast-enhanced MRI of the lumbar spine may also be a useful screening procedure. The next step is a lumbar puncture for CSF cytology. A large CSF volume, preferably 10 mL, should be rapidly processed by the pathology laboratory. If cytology is negative, a second sample should be taken. The sensitivity of the procedure may be increased by using additional techniques, including flow cytometry, or immunohistochemistry. Additional lumbar punctures, or alternatively, a cisternal puncture may be considered to improve diagnostic yield.

Acknowledgment

The author wishes to express her gratitude to Dr H.G. de Bruin, radiologist in the Daniel den Hoed Cancer Center / Erasmus Medical Center Rotterdam, The Netherlands, for providing the images.

REFERENCES

1. Posner, J. B. and Chernik, N. L. Intracranial metastases from systemic cancer. Schoenberg, B. S. 579-592. 1978. New York, Raven Press. Advances in Neurology.
2. Olson ME, Chernik NL, Posner JB. Infiltration of leptomeninges by systemic cancer clinical and pathologic study. Arch Neurol 1974; 30:122-37.
3. Wasserstrom WR, Glass JP, Posner JB. Diagnosis and Treatment of leptomeningeal metastases from solid tumors - experience with 90 patients. Cancer 1982; 49:759-72.
4. Haaxma-Reiche, H. Neurological complications of leukemia. Vecht, C. J. (25 (69)), 233-260. 1997. Elsevier Science B.V. Handbook of Clinical Neurology: Neuro-Oncology, Part III.
5. Singh SK, Agris JM, Leeds NE, Ginsberg LE. Intracranial leptomeningeal metastases: Comparison of depiction at FLAIR and contrast-enhanced MR imaging. Radiology 2000; 217:50-3.
6. Singh SK, Leeds NE, Ginsberg LE. MR imaging of leptomeningeal metastases: Comparison of three sequences. Am J Neuroradiol 2002; 23:817-21.

7. Bigner SH, Johnston WW. The diagnostic challenge of tumors manifested initially by the shedding of cells into cerebrospinal fluid. Acta Cytologica 1984; 28:29-36.
8. Glass JP, Melamed M, Chernik NL, Posner JB. Malignant-Cells in cerebrospinal Fluid (CSF) - Meaning of a positive CSF cytology. Neurology 1979; 29:1369-75.
9. Glantz MJ, Cole BF, Glantz LK, Cobb J, Mills P, Lekos A et al. Cerebrospinal fluid cytology in patients with cancer - Minimizing false-negative results. Cancer 1998; 82:733-9.
10. Chamberlain MC. Cytologically negative carcinomatous meningitis: Usefulness of CSF biochemical markers. Neurology 1998; 50:1173-5.
11. van Oostenbrugge RJ, Twijnstra A. Presenting features and value of diagnostic procedures in leptomeningeal metastases. Neurology 1999; 53:382-5.
12. Nakagawa H, Murasawa A, Kubo S, Nakajima S, Nakajima Y, Izumoto S et al. Diagnosis and treatment of patients with meningeal carcinomatosis. J Neuro-Oncol 1992; 13:81-9.
13. Twijnstra A, Devisser BWO, Vanzanten AP. Diagnosis of leptomeningeal metastasis. Clin Neurol Neurosurg 1987; 89:79-85.
14. Rosen ST, Aisner J, Makuch RW, Matthews MJ, Ihde DC, Whitacre M et al. Carcinomatous leptomeningitis in small cell lung cancer - A clinicopathologic review of the National Cancer Institute Experience. Medicine 1982; 61:45-53.
15. Theodore WH, Gendelman S. Meningeal carcinomatosis. Arch Neurol 1981; 38:696-9.
16. Recht L, Straus DJ, Cirrincione C, Thaler HT, Posner JB. Central nervous system metastases from non-Hodgkins lymphoma - treatment and prophylaxis. Am J Med 1988; 84:425-35.
17. Surapaneni UR, Cortes JE, Thomas D, O'Brien S, Giles FJ, Koller C et al. Central nervous system relapse in adults with acute lymphoblastic leukemia. Cancer 2002; 94:773-9.
18. van Besien K, Ha CS, Murphy S, McLaughlin P, Rodriguez A, Amin K et al. Risk factors, treatment, and outcome of central nervous system recurrence in adults with intermediate-grade and immunoblastic lymphoma. Blood 1998; 91:1178-84.
19. Yap HY, Yap BS, Tashima CK, Distefano A, Blumenschein GR. Meningeal carcinomatosis in breast cancer. Cancer 1978; 42:283-6.
20. Boogerd W, Hart AAM, Vandersande JJ, Engelsman E. Meningeal Carcinomatosis in breast cancer - prognostic factors and influence of treatment. Cancer 1991; 67:1685-95.
21. Chamberlain MC, Kormanik P. Carcinoma meningitis secondary to non-small cell lung cancer - combined modality therapy. Arch Neurol 1998; 55:506-12.
22. Burger B, Zimmermann M, Mann G, Kuhl J, Loning L, Reihm H et al. Diagnostic cerebrospinal fluid examination in children with acute lymphoblastic leukemia: Significance of low leukocyte counts with blasts or traumatic lumbar puncture. J Clin Oncol 2003; 21:184-8.
23. Mastrangelo R, Poplack D, Bleyer A, Riccardi R, Sather H, Dangio G. Report and recommendations of the Rome Workshop concerning poor prognosis acute lymphoblastic-leukemia in children - Biologic bases for staging, stratification, and treatment. Med Ped Oncol 1986; 14:191-4.
24. Abbott BL, Rubnitz JE, Tong X, Srivastava DK, Pui CH, Ribeiro RC et al. Clinical significance of central nervous system involvement at diagnosis of pediatric acute myeloid leukemia: a single institution's experience. Leukemia 2003; 17:2090-6.
25. Sariban E, Edwards B, Janus C, Magrath I. Central nervous system involvement in American Burkitts lymphoma. J Clin Oncol 1983; 1:677-81.
26. Gururangan S, Sposto R, Cairo MS, Meadows AT, Finlay JL. Outcome of CNS disease at diagnosis in disseminated small noncleaved-cell lymphoma and B-cell leukemia: A Children's Cancer Group study. J Clin Oncol 2000; 18:2017-25.
27. Haddy TB, Adde MA, Magrath IT. CNS involvement in small non-cleaved cell lymphoma - Is CNS disease per se a poor prognostic sign. J Clin Oncol 1991; 9:1973-82.
28. Sandlund JT, Murphy SB, Santana VM, Behm F, Jones D, Berard CW et al. CNS involvement in children with newly diagnosed non-Hodgkin's lymphoma. J Clin Oncol

2000; 18:3018-24.
29. Abrey LE, Rosenblum MK, DeAngelis LM. Sarcoidosis of the cauda equina mimicking leptomeningeal malignancy. J Neuro-Oncol 1998; 39:261-5.
30. Sze G. Leptomeningeal tumor: the "Plain vanilla" approach remains the best. Am J Neuroradiol 2002; 23:745-6.
31. Tsukada Y, Fouad A, Pickren JW, Lane WW. Central nervous system metastasis from breast carcinoma - autopsy study. Cancer 1983; 52:2349-54.
32. Amer MH, Alsarraf M, Baker LH, Vaitkevicius VK. Malignant melanoma and central nervous system metastases - incidence, diagnosis, treatment and survival. Cancer 1978; 42:660-8.
33. Jayson GC, Howell A, Harris M, Morgenstern G, Chang J, Ryder WD. Carcinomatous meningitis in patients with breast cancer - an aggressive disease variant. Cancer 1994; 74:3135-41.
34. Lee JL, Kang YK, Kim TW, Chang HM, Lee GW, Ryu MH et al. Leptomeningeal carcinomatosis in gastric cancer. J Neuro-Oncol 2004; 66:167-74.
35. Smith DB, Howell A, Harris M, Bramwell VHC, Sellwood RA. Carcinomatous meningitis associated with infiltrating lobular carcinoma of the breast. Eur J Surg Oncol 1985; 11:33-6.
36. Kantarjian HM, O'Brien S, Smith TL, Cortes J, Giles FJ, Beran M et al. Results of treatment with Hyper-CVAD, a dose-intensive regimen, in adult acute lymphocytic leukemia. J Clin Oncol 2000; 18:547-61.
37. Pui CH, Dahl GV, Kalwinsky DK, Look AT, Mirro J, Dodge RK et al. Central nervous system leukemia in children with acute non-lymphoblastic leukemia. Blood 1985; 66:1062-7.
38. Dusenbery KE, Howells WB, Arthur DC, Alonzo T, Lee JW, Kobrinsky N et al. Extramedullary leukemia in children with newly diagnosed acute myeloid leukemia - A report from the children's cancer group. J Ped Hematol Oncol 2003; 25:760-8.
39. Peterson BA, Brunning RD, Bloomfield CD, Hurd DD, Gau JA, Peng GT et al. Central nervous system involvement in acute non-lymphocytic leukemia - A prospective study of adults in remission. Am J Med 1987; 83:464-70.
40. Colovic N, Bogdanovic A, Miljic P, Jankovic G, Colovic M. Central nervous system relapse in acute promyelocytic leukemia. Am J Hematol 2002; 71:60-1.
41. Breccia M, Carmosino I, Diverio D, De Santis S, De Propris MS, Romano A et al. Early detection of meningeal localization in acute promyelocytic leukaemia patients with high presenting leucocyte count. Br J Haematol 2003; 120:266-70.
42. Cramer SC, Glaspy JA, Efird JT, Louis DN. Chronic lymphocytic leukemia and the central nervous system: A clinical and pathological study. Neurology 1996; 46:19-25.
43. Akintola-Ogunremi O, Whitney C, Mathur SC, Finch CN. Chronic lymphocytic leukemia presenting with symptomatic central nervous system involvement. Ann Hematol 2002; 81:402-4.
44. Cavanna L, Invernizzi R, Berte R, Vallisa D, Buscarini L. Meningeal involvement in multiple myeloma - Report of a case with cytologic and immunocytochemical diagnosis. Acta Cytologica 1996; 40:571-5.
45. Evans LS, Hancock BW. Non-Hodgkin lymphoma. Lancet 2003; 362:139-46.
46. van den Bent, M. J. Neurological complications of systemic lymphoma. Vecht, C. J. 261-287. 1997. Elsevier Science B.V. Handbook of Clinical Neurology; Neuro-Oncology, Part III.
47. Buckstein R, Lim W, Franssen E, Imrie KL. CNS prophylaxis and treatment in non-Hodgkin's lymphoma: Variation in practice and lessons from the literature. Leukemia Lymphoma 2003; 44:955-62.
48. Hoelzer, D. and Gokbuget, N. Treatment of lymphoblastic lymphoma in adults. Best Prac Res Clin Haematol 2003; 15:713-728.
49. Ersboll J, Schultz HB, Thomsen BLR, Keiding N, Nissen NI. Meningeal involvement in non-Hodgkin's lymphoma: Symptoms, incidence, risk factors and treatment. Scand J Haematol 1985; 35:478-96.

50. Haioun C, Besson C, Lepage E, Simon D, Rose C, Tilly H et al. Incidence and rise factors of central nervous system (CNS) relapse in histologically aggressive non-Hodgkin's lymphoma (NHL) uniformly treated and receiving prophylaxis for CNS a GELA study on 974 patients. Blood 1999; 94:522A.
51. Zucca E, Conconi A, Mughal TI, Sarris AH, Seymour JF, Vitolo U et al. Patterns of outcome and prognostic factors in primary large-cell lymphoma of the testis in a survey by the International Extranodal Lymphoma Study Group. J Clin Oncol 2003; 21:20-7.
52. Kaufman DK, Habermann TM, Kurtin PJ, Oneill BP. Neurological complications of peripheral and cutaneous T-cell lymphomas. Annals of Neurology 1994; 36:625-9.
53. Teshima T, Akashi K, Shibuya T, Taniguchi S, Okamura T, Harada M et al. Central nervous system involvement in adult T-cell leukemia lymphoma. Cancer 1990; 65:327-32.
54. Balmaceda C, Gaynor JJ, Sun M, Gluck JT, DeAngelis LM. Leptomeningeal tumor in primary central nervous system lymphoma - recognition, significance, and implications. Ann Neurol 1995; 38:202-9.
55. Robertson PL, Zeltzer PM, Boyett JM, Rorke LB, Allen JC, Geyer JR et al. Survival and prognostic factors following radiation therapy and chemotherapy for ependymomas in children: a report of the Children's Cancer Group. J Neurosurg 1998; 88:695-703.
56. Saito R, Kumabe T, Jokura H, Shirane R, Yoshimoto T. Symptomatic spinal dissemination of malignant astrocytoma. J Neuro-Oncol 2003; 61:227-35.
57. Zeltzer PM, Boyett JM, Finlay JL, Albright AL, Rorke LB, Milstein JM et al. Metastasis stage, adjuvant treatment, and residual tumor are prognostic factors for medulloblastoma in children: Conclusions from the Children's Cancer Group 921 randomized phase III study. J Clin Oncol 1999; 17:832-45.
58. Kortmann RD, Kuhl J, Timmermann B, Mittler U, Urban C, Budach V et al. Postoperative neoadjuvant chemotherapy before radiotherapy as compared to immediate radiotherapy followed by maintenance chemotherapy in the treatment of medulloblastoma in childhood: Results of the German prospective randomized trial HIT '91. Int J Radiat Oncol Biol Phys 2000; 46:269-79.
59. Fouladi M, Gajjar A, Boyett JM, Walter AW, Thompson SJ, Merchant TE et al. Comparison of CSF cytology and spinal magnetic resonance imaging in the detection of leptomeningeal disease in pediatric medulloblastoma or primitive neuroectodermal tumor. J Clin Oncol 1999; 17:3234-7.
60. DeAngelis LM. Current diagnosis and treatment of leptomeningeal metastasis. J Neuro-Oncol 1998; 38:245-52.
61. Posner, J. B. Leptomeningeal metastases in Neurologic Complications of Cancer. 1st, 143-171. 1995. Philadelphia, F.A. Davis Company. Contemporary Neurology Series vol 45.
62. Grossman SA, Krabak MJ. Leptomeningeal carcinomatosis. Cancer Treat Rev 1999; 25:103-19.
63. Chamberlain MC. Leptomeningeal metastases: A review of evaluation and treatment. J Neuro-Oncol 1998; 37:271-84.
64. Mackintosh FR, Colby TV, Podolsky WJ, Burke JS, Hoppe RT, Rosenfelt FP et al. Central nervous system involvement in non-Hodgkins lymphoma - An analysis of 105 cases. Cancer 1982; 49:586-95.
65. Hitchins RN, Bell DR, Woods RL, Levi JA. A prospective randomized trial of single-agent versus combination chemotherapy in meningeal carcinomatosis. J Clin Oncol 1987; 5:1655-62.
66. Kaplan JG, Desouza TG, Farkash A, Shafran B, Pack D, Rehman F et al. Leptomeningeal metastases - comparison of clinical features and laboratory data of solid tumors, lymphomas and leukemias. J Neuro-Oncol 1990; 9:225-9.
67. Balm M, Hammack J. Leptomeningeal carcinomatosis - Presenting features and prognostic factors. Arch Neurol 1996; 53:626-32.
68. Pedersen AG, Olsen J, Nasiell M. Cerebrospinal fluid cytology diagnosis of meningeal carcinomatosis in patients with small cell carcinoma of the lung - A study of interobserver and intraobserver variability. Acta Cytologica 1986; 30:648-52.

69. Little JR, Dale AJD, Okazaki H. meningeal carcinomatosis - clinical manifestations. Arch Neurol 1974; 30:138-43.
70. Fizazi K, Asselain B, VincentSalomon A, Jouve M, Dieras V, Palangie T et al. Meningeal carcinomatosis in patients with breast carcinoma - Clinical features, prognostic factors, and results of a high-dose intrathecal methotrexate regimen. Cancer 1996; 77:1315-23.
71. Straathof CSM, de Bruin HG, Dippel DWJ, Vecht CJ. The diagnostic accuracy of magnetic resonance imaging and cerebrospinal fluid cytology in leptomeningeal metastasis. J Neurol 1999; 246:810-4.
72. Dux R, Kindlerrohrborn A, Annas M, Faustmann P, Lennartz K, Zimmermann CW. A standardized protocol for flow cytometric analysis of cells isolated from cerebrospinal fluid. J Neurol Sci 1994; 121:74-8.
73. van Oostenbrugge RJ, Hopman AHN, Lenders MH, van Heerde P, Arends JW, Ramaekers FCS et al. Detection of malignant cells in cerebrospinal fluid using fluorescence in situ hybridization. J Neuropathol Exp Neurol 1997; 56:743-8.
74. Roma AA, Garcia A, Avagnina A, Rescia C, Elsner B. Lymphoid and myeloid neoplasms involving cerebrospinal fluid: Comparison of morphologic examination and immunophenotyping by flow cytometry. Diag Cytopathol 2002; 27:271-5.
75. Hovestadt A, Henzenlogmans SC, Vecht CJ. Immunohistochemical analysis of the cerebrospinal fluid for carcinomatous and lymphomatous leptomeningitis. Br J Cancer 1990; 62:653-4.
76. Boogerd W, Vroom TM, Vanheerde P, Delariviere GB, Peterse JL, Vandersande JJ. CSF cytology versus immunocytochemistry in meningeal carcinomatosis. J Neurol Neurosurg Psychiatry 1988; 51:142-5.
77. Jorda M, Ganjei-Azar P, Nadji M. Cytologic characteristics of meningeal carcinomatosis - Increased diagnostic accuracy using carcinoembryonic antigen and epithelial membrane antigen immunocytochemistry. Arch Neurol 1998; 55:181-4.
78. Kranz BR. Detection of rare malignant cells and their apoptotic fragments in cerebrospinal fluid. Lancet 2000; 356:1242-4.
79. de Haas V, Vet RJWM, Verhagen OJHM, Kroes W, van den Berg H, van der Schoot CE. Early detection of central nervous system relapse by polymerase chain reaction in children with B-precursor acute lymphoblastic leukemia. Ann Hematol 2002; 81:59-61.
80. Galoin S, Daste G, Apoil PA, Chollet F, Roda D, Blancher A et al. Polymerase chain reaction on cerebrospinal fluid cells in the detection of leptomeningeal involvement by B-cell lymphoma and leukaemia: a novel strategy and its implications. Br J Haematol 1997; 99:122-30.
81. Rhodes CH, Glantz MJ, Glantz L, Lekos A, Sorenson GD, Honsinger C et al. A comparison of polymerase chain reaction examination of cerebrospinal fluid and conventional cytology in the diagnosis of lymphomatous meningitis. Cancer 1996; 77:543-8.
82. Twijnstra A, Vanzanten AP, Nooyen WJ, Devisser BWO. Sensitivity and specificity of single and combined tumor markers in the diagnosis of leptomeningeal metastasis from breast cancer. J Neurol Neurosurg Psychiatry 1986; 49:1246-50.
83. Fleisher M, Wasserstrom WR, Schold SC, Schwartz MK, Posner JB. Lactic dehydrogenase isoenzymes in the cerebrospinal fluid of patients with systemic cancer. Cancer 1981; 47:2654-9.
84. van den Bent MJ, Lamers CHJ, 't Veer MB, Smitt PAES, Bolhuis RLH, Gratama JW. Increased levels of soluble CD27 in the cerebrospinal fluid are not diagnostic for leptomeningeal involvement by lymphoid malignancies. Ann Hematol 2002; 81:187-91.
85. Rogers LR, Duchesneau PM, Nunez C, Fishleder AJ, Weick JK, Bauer LJ et al. Comparison of cisternal and lumbar CSF examination in leptomeningeal metastasis. Neurology 1992; 42:1239-41.
86. Chamberlain MC, Kormanik PA, Glantz MJ. A comparison between ventricular and lumbar cerebrospinal fluid cytology in adult patients with leptomeningeal metastases. Neuro-Oncol 2001; 3:42-5.

87. Gajjar A, Fouladi M, Walter AW, Thompson SJ, Reardon DA, Merchant TE et al. Comparison of lumbar and shunt cerebrospinal fluid specimens for cytologic detection of leptomeningeal disease in pediatric patients with brain tumors. J Clin Oncol 1999; 17:1825-8.
88. Freilich RJ, Krol G, DeAngelis LM. Neuroimaging and cerebrospinal fluid cytology in the diagnosis of leptomeningeal metastasis. Ann Neurol 1995; 38:51-7.
89. Zeiser R, Burger JA, Bley TA, Windfuhr-Blum M, Schulte-Monting J, Behringer DM. Clinical follow-up indicates differential accuracy of magnetic resonance imaging and immunocytology of the cerebral spinal fluid for the diagnosis of neoplastic meningitis - a single centre experience. Br J Haematol 2004; 124:762-8.
90. Chamberlain MC. Comparative spine imaging in leptomeningeal metastases. J Neuro-Oncol 1995; 23:233-8.
91. Yousem DM, Patrone PM, Grossman RI. Leptomeningeal metastases - MR evaluation. J Comp Assis Tomogr 1990; 14:255-61.
92. Gomori JM, Heching N, Siegal T. Leptomeningeal metastases: Evaluation by gadolinium enhanced spinal magnetic resonance imaging. J Neuro-Oncol 1998; 36:55-60.
93. Hsia AW, Katz JS, Hancock SL, Peterson K. Post-irradiation polyradiculopathy mimics leptomeningeal tumor on MRI. *Neurology* 2003; 60:1694-6.
94. Jeha LE, Sila CA, Lederman RJ, Prayson RA, Isada CM, Gordon SM. West Nile virus infection - A new acute paralytic illness. Neurology 2003; 61:55-9.
95. Schumacher M, Orszagh M. Imaging techniques in neoplastic meningiosis. J Neuro-Oncol 1998; 38:111-20.
96. Pannullo SC, Reich JB, Krol G, Deck MDF, Posner JB. MRI changes in intracranial hypotension. Neurology 1993; 43:919-26.

Chapter 3

LEPTOMENINGEAL METASTASES FROM SOLID TUMORS (MENINGEAL CARCINOMATOSIS)

Michiko Kimura Bruno, M.D., Jeffrey Raizer, M.D.
Northwestern University, 710 North Lake Shore Drive, Chicago, Ill.

Abstract: Leptomeningeal metastases (LM) are increasingly recognized as a devastating complication of solid tumors. Improved treatment of primary malignancy and advances in diagnostic imaging have led to an apparent increase in the number of patients diagnosed with LM. Unfortunately, therapeutic options remain limited. Radiotherapy is used to treat bulky tumor and provide symptomatic relief. Intrathecal chemotherapy benefits a selected subset of patients. The challenge to the future is to delineate the molecular mechanisms underlying LM and to develop novel therapeutic or prophylactic modalities to combat LM.

Key Words: Leptomeningeal metastases; breast cancer; lung cancer; solid tumors; intrathecal chemotherapy

1. INTRODUCTION

Leptomeningeal metastases (LM) from solid tumors remain a difficult complication for oncologists and neurologists due to the high incidence of neurological morbidity and mortality. Early detection of LM is important for both prognostic and therapeutic reasons. LM was first recognized by Eberth[35] and felt to be a rare complication of solid tumors; recently, its incidence appears to be increasing.[33,55,90] One reason for this increase is that most chemotherapeutic agents or regimens for systemic malignancies do not penetrate the blood-brain barrier (BBB) to any significant degree; therefore, malignant cells within the nervous system may proliferate despite patients having a systemic response or remission of their cancer.[12,40] Secondly, awareness of this complication and the ability of magnetic resonance imaging (MRI) to diagnose LM have also lead to earlier diagnosis and contributed to the increased incidence.

2. EPIDEMIOLOGY

The incidence of LM among all cancer patients is as high as 8%.[51,90] However, no recent studies have re-evaluated the overall incidence. Autopsy data show that 19% of all cancer patients develop LM, 40% of whom had a negative cerebrospinal fluid (CSF) cytology prior to death.[51,91]

LM from solid tumors typically occurs with advanced stage disease when patients have diffuse systemic metastases. Twenty percent of patients have isolated LM while approximately 30% of patients with LM have concomitant brain or epidural metastases.[85,134] In large cancer centers, LM was found to be the initial manifestation of cancer in 6-21% of patients.[9,85,134]

Any solid tumor can metastasize to the leptomeninges; however, melanoma, lung, and breast cancer have the highest predilection for the leptomeninges. Cancers that are less likely to metastasize to the leptomeninges include squamous cell cancers of the head and neck, ovarian cancer and thyroid cancer (Table 1).

Table 1: Frequency of LM by solid tumor type[85,134]

Cancer	Frequency
Breast	51.0 %
Lung:	
Small-Cell	7.1 %
Non-small cell	17.0 %
Melanoma	13.0 %
GU	4.8 %
GI	1.6 %
Head/Neck	1.6 %
Unknown primary	2.4 %
Other	1.6 %

The incidence of LM in patients with small cell lung cancer is between 9-25%.[3,5,8,99] The incidence appears to increase with length of survival from 0.5% at cancer diagnosis to 25% after three years.[99] Aroney et al reported that 42 % of patients who relapsed after initial treatment did so in the leptomeninges; this being the only site of relapse in 27 %.[5] For patients with small cell lung cancer and limited stage disease, prophylactic cranial radiotherapy (RT) is recommended to prevent brain metastases;[6] however, this does not prevent leptomeningeal spread.[6,8] Although the exact incidence of LM among patients with non-small cell lung cancer has not been reported, it is estimated that LM from non-small cell lung cancer comprises 10 to 19 % of all LM.[9,85,134]

The incidence of LM from breast cancer is between 2-8 % and is usually associated with concurrent brain or epidural metastasis.[51,60,122,137] Patients who are estrogen-receptor negative have a higher incidence of LM.[34]

The incidence of LM from melanoma is about 23%.[4] The exact incidence in genitourinary (GU) cancers (renal, bladder and prostate) is not reported but 6 % of all LM patients have GU malignancies, and the incidence rate may be increasing.[12,32,74,115,134] Gastrointestinal (GI) cancers were once believed to be a major cause of LM but are now rarely encountered.[38] LM from gynecological cancers (ovarian, cervical, and fallopian tube adenocarcinoma) and head and neck cancers are also seen.[1, 7, 95, 128] Rare solid tumors that metastasize to the leptomeninges include thyroid cancer,[10] retinoblastoma,[55] neuroblastoma,[65] neuroendocrine tumors,[36] carcinoid,[79] sarcoma,[62, 134] and squamous cell of the skin or larynx.[11,120,140]

3. PATHOPHYSIOLOGY

There are multiple mechanisms by which tumor cells can disseminate into the subarachnoid spaces. Once the tumor cells gain access to the CSF, there is direct communication with the entire subarachnoid space. Tumor cells are carried by bulk flow, with most deposits occurring at the base of the skull or spine.

Tumor cells can hematogenously spread to involve the brain parenchyma or choroid plexus. Once implanted they may rupture seeding the leptomeninges with micrometastases. However, not all patients have concomitant CNS or choroid plexus metastases suggesting that there must be other mechanisms. Detailed pathological review has failed to demonstrate tumor cells within the lumen of the leptomeningeal arterial vasculature; therefore, hematogenous spread through leptomeningeal arteries is unlikely.[65] In leukemia, malignant cells enter the subarachnoid space via thin-walled microscopic veins in the arachnoid membrane and seed the meninges.[92] Malignant cells also extend into the Virchow-Robin space. Similar mechanisms may also hold true for solid tumors.

Direct extension is a second mechanism by which invasion into the subarachnoid space occurs. This can occur by paravertebral spread along the cranial or spinal nerve roots, invasion of the perineural spaces by the primary focus, cervical lymph nodes communicating directly with the subarachnoid space, and tumor growth into the subdural space. Extension from Batson's plexus and perivenous spread from bone marrow metastases has also been proposed.[55] Posterior fossa craniotomies for resection of cerebellar metastases appear to be a risk factor for the development of LM, likely from the proximity of the lesion to the CSF spaces.[83, 129]

4. CLINICAL MANIFESTATION

Multifocal neurologic signs and symptoms are the hallmark of LM. Symptoms can be divided into CNS, cranial neuropathies or spinal/radicular (Table 2). The mechanisms in which LM cause neurological signs and symptoms include obstruction of CSF flow or drainage with resultant increased intracranial pressure (ICP), meningeal irritation, or focal signs from local invasion or irritation of the brain, cranial nerves, spinal cord or spinal nerves. LM can cause cerebral infarction from a cerebral vasculopathy; changes in brain metabolism and reduction in cerebral blood flow may cause a diffuse encephalopathy.[62, 106] Isolated neurologic symptoms occur in 30-53 % of patients with LM,[9, 61, 85, 131, 135, 137] with CNS[85] and spinal/radicular[61] the most common. Multifocal involvement is seen in 40-80 % of cases.[9, 61, 85, 131, 135 137] In one study, a combination of two sites was seen in 47 % of cases (CNS 29 %, CNS and spinal/radicular 10%, and spinal/radicular 8%) and involvement of all levels was seen in 13% of patients.[137] Historically, it has been said that signs are much more significant than symptoms;[85] for example, a patient may complain of headache, but on examination has facial weakness, dorsiflexor weakness and an absent deep tendon reflex.

Table 2. Symptoms and signs of Leptomeningeal Metastases[9, 85, 135, 137]

Symptoms	%	Signs	%
CNS			
Headache	28-50		
MS change	25-34	Altered mental status	27-50
Nausea/vomiting	12-34	Upper motor neuron weakness	9-26
Gait	46		
Episodic LOC	6-18		
Dizziness	2		
Cranial nerve			
Diplopia	8-20	II	
Visual loss	8	Papilledema	12
Dysarthria/dysphagia	2-7	Optic atrophy	2
Hearing loss	6	III, IV, VI	24-30

Table 2. (Continued)

		V	6- 12
		VII	10-25
		VIII	7-20
		IX,X	8-13
		XI	3
		XII	2-8
Spinal/radicular			
Neck/back pain	18	Weakness	78
Radicular pain	12	Reflex asymmetry	60
Paresthesia	10-25	Sensory loss	50
Weakness	22-34	Straight leg raise	12
Bowel/bladder	2-18	Decreased rectal tone	5
		Nuchal rigidity	13-16

4.1 Central nervous system signs and symptoms

Headache is seen in approximately 50 % of patients with LM and is often associated with nausea, vomiting or lightheadedness. Meningismus and nuchal rigidity are seen in about 15 % of patients. Other common symptoms include an alteration in mental status and gait disturbances. Episodic loss of consciousness may be due to seizures from cortical irritation or plateau waves when there is elevated ICP, even in the absence of significant hydrocephalus. Less frequent presentations include focal neurological deficits, diabetes insipidus, cerebral salt wasting, cerebral infarction, non-convulsive status epilepticus, central hypoventilation and psychiatric manifestations.[20, 69, 87, 118, 136]

4.2 Cranial neuropathies

Patients may complain of diplopia, numbness, visual loss, hearing loss or vertigo.[137] Less commonly, they can have decreased taste, dysarthria, swallowing difficulty, hoarseness or glossopharyngeal neuralgia.[111] LM from solid tumors more commonly affects the oculomotor nerves, whereas the facial nerves are more affected in hematological malignancies.[137] Nevertheless, isolated peripheral facial nerve palsy in cancer patients should not be dismissed as Bell's palsy, especially if it does not spontaneously resolve. The differential diagnosis of cranial neuropathies in cancer patients include base of skull metastasis, soft tissue invasion, infiltration of extra cranial nerve structures, or infection.

4.3 Spinal signs and symptoms

More than 50 % of patients with LM have spinal symptoms. The cauda equina is a common site of nodular formation. Pain is a common complaint and is the presenting symptom in as many as 76% of patients.[87] Pain is usually in the lower back, worse in a supine position and occurs in the morning. Patients can have segmental or diffuse lower extremity weakness, radicular pain, paresthesias, generalized or focal sensory loss, leg cramps, and bowel or bladder dysfunction. Loss of deep tendon reflexes can be found in 70% patients, although cancer patients frequently have this finding from previous chemotherapy.[135, 137] Occasionally, patients with cauda equina LM present with flaccid paraparesis mimicking epidural cord compression. An unusual presentation mimicking the Miller-Fisher variant of Guillain-Barré syndrome has been reported.[56]

5. DIAGNOSIS

5.1 Cerebrospinal fluid (CSF)

Examination of the CSF for malignant cells is the gold standard for the diagnosis of LM; however, with the advent of MRI the diagnoses can often be made non-invasively. Unfortunately, the sensitivity of cytology on the initial CSF is only about 50 %; however, less than 5% of patients have a completely normal CSF profile Table 3). [51, 85, 90, 135]

Table 3: CSF Findings in Leptomeningeal Metastases [48, 55, 61, 135]

	Initial	Subsequent
Positive cytology	45-75 %	90 %
Elevated pressure	44-50 %	64 %
Elevated protein	73-86 %	80 %
Low glucose	20-56 %	37 %
Elevated WBC	51-79 %	65 %
Completely normal profile	2-5 %	1 %

The low initial sensitivity of cytologic examination may be attributed to the fact that tumor cells adhere to the meninges with few free-floating cells resulting in negative cytology. Increasing the CSF volume (10-20 cc), examining the specimen as soon as possible, and performing serial lumbar punctures (LP) may increase the diagnostic yield. If the specimen is delivered within minutes it may be examined without fixation, but routinely it is fixed in an equal volume of fixate. A recent review suggests that two LPs may be sufficient to achieve a sensitivity of 90 %.[48]

The CSF cytology results may vary if the sample is obtained from Ommaya reservoir as opposed to LP.[55,90] The sensitivity may be dependent upon the localization of clinical symptoms. When only cranial signs or symptoms are present, the ventricular CSF is nearly three times more likely to be positive than lumbar, whereas when only spinal signs or symptoms were present, the lumbar CSF is nearly three times more likely to be positive than the ventricular CSF.[27] CSF is also more likely to be positive when LM is more disseminated than when it is focal.[51] Cisternal puncture is an alternative way to collect CSF and may be positive even when the fluid is negative.[97] This is done by a lateral cervical puncture at the C2 level under fluoroscopic visualization. It may be more likely to yield a positive cytology when cranial signs and symptoms present. When CSF remains negative, other abnormalities of the CSF may aid in the diagnosis of LM.

Elevated CSF pressure is seen in approximately 50 % of patients with LM. Obstruction of the arachnoid granulations by malignant cells is the likely cause of increased pressure which can ultimately lead to hydrocephalus. However, there are other etiologies that can elevate CSF pressure in cancer patients including cerebral sinus thrombosis,[94] or an increase in systemic venous pressure due to compression or obstruction of superior vena cava or jugular vein.

The white blood cell count is elevated in approximately 50% of patients. Red blood cells or xanthochromia can be seen from bleeding due to LM, especially with melanoma.[90] Elevated CSF protein is seen in approximately 70-85% of patients with LM but is a non-specific finding. Low glucose is seen in 40% of patients with LM; it is a relatively specific finding for this condition, especially when less than 10. Tuberculous and bacterial meningitis can have a low glucose and need to be excluded. A normal CSF glucose level in a diabetic patient may indicate hypoglycorrhachia. The mechanism of hypoglycorrhachia is unclear but may be due to diminished carrier-mediated transport of glucose across the BBB or glucose metabolism by malignant and reactive cells.[90]

Used in the appropriate clinical setting, certain biochemical markers in the CSF can aid in the diagnosis of LM. Metastases outside the leptomeninges, such as parenchyma brain metastases, do not usually elevate these markers.[133] They can also be helpful in monitoring disease activity or response to treatment.[103] Unfortunately, the sensitivity of these markers is generally low, the normal values for certain markers are unknown, and some are investigational.

Specific markers include carcinoembryonic antigen (CEA) found in adenocarcinomas of the lung, breast, colon and bladder cancer,[39, 103, 133] alpha-fetoprotein (AFP) found in teratocarcinoma, yolk sac tumor, endodermal sinus tumor and embryonal carcinoma, and beta-human chorionic gonadotropin (b-HCG) found in choriocarcinoma, embryonal carcinoma and germ-cell tumors. [133] Five- hydroxyindole acetic acid (5-HIAA) is a substance found in normal CSF, but if grossly elevated may be helpful in making the diagnosis of carcinoid.[79] Other specific markers include prostate specific antigen (PSA) in prostate cancer,[74] alkaline phosphatase level and CA 19-9 in lung cancer,[66,102] CA 125 in ovarian cancer,[90] CA 15-3 in breast cancer, [90] and gastrin releasing peptide in small cell carcinoma. [21]

In order to interpret the results of these markers in CSF, serum levels should be obtained simultaneously because high serum levels can diffuse into the CSF. In the case of CEA, levels greater than 1 % of serum CEA in the spinal fluid suggests LM.[103]

Nonspecific markers include beta-glucuronidase,[39, 103, 126, 127, 133] LDH isoenzyme-5,[39, 126, 127] beta 2-microglobulin,[126, 127] myelin basic protein,[107] ferritin,[140] an epithelial glycoprotein HMFG1 antigen,[76] and tumor necrosis factor-alpha[81]. These nonspecific markers can be elevated in CNS processes other than LM including bacterial meningitis and stroke, but in combination may increase diagnostic accuracy of LM.[127]. Recently, vascular endothelial growth factor (VEGF), a potent promoter of tumor angiogenesis, was found to be significantly elevated in patients with LM but not in the CSF of patients in the control group.[113] Certain matrix metalloproteinase (MMP) profiles have been shown to correlate with LM compared to patients with brain metastases, primary brain tumors, and controls; patients with LM have activation of MMP-2 and -9.[42] Elevation of cathepsin B and H and decreased cystatin C in CSF was found in the CSF of patients with LM but not in controls, suggesting that this may be another diagnostic marker.[78] In general, levels of all of these markers are lower in ventricular than in lumbar fluid. [103]

Newer techniques may assist the diagnosis of LM from solid tumors. In flow cytometry, molecular markers and chromosomal analysis may detect abnormalities suggesting tumor cells. Polymerase chain reaction (PCR) analysis of known genetic alterations may increase the diagnostic yield of CSF studies.[29, 44,117] Florescence in situ hybridization (FISH) detects the chromosomal aberrations in the interphase nucleus.[130, 132] One study tested the aneusomy of chromosome 1, which is frequently involved in carcinogenesis of solid tumors, and found a better correlation with neurologic status and accurate diagnosis of LM.[132]

5.2 Computed tomography scan (CT) and magnetic resonance imaging (MRI)

MRI has dramatically increased the diagnostic yield of LM.[41] The sensitivity of MRI is approximately 75% with a specificity of 77 %.[31,114]

Linear or nodular enhancement can be seen on the surface of the cerebrum or within the cerebellar folia, basal cisterns, cranial or spinal nerves and nerve roots after administration of gadolinium. Diffuse leptomeningeal enhancement can be seen, but is not as sensitive as focal dural enhancement which may be reactive from base of skull metastasis or from intracranial hypotension, typically after LP.[96] Therefore, contrast enhanced MRI should be performed before LP. Other processes that may mimic LM include neurosarcoidosis,[2] chronic meningitis or Guillain-Barré syndrome.[52]

Fluid-attenuated inversion recovery (FLAIR) sequences are somewhat less sensitive than T_1 gadolinium images, but may detect small abnormalities as bright signals within the subarachnoid space often missed with gadolinium.[109] Contrast-enhanced FLAIR may further improve the sensitivity.[71] A comparison of these three techniques suggests that contrast enhanced T1 images remain the most accurate with a sensitivity of 59% and specificity of 93%, compared to unenhanced FLAIR of 12% and 93%, enhanced FLAIR of 41% and 88%, respectively. Using all three sequences the sensitivity is 65%.[110]

CT is not as sensitive as MRI, although nodular enhancement may be seen in some cases. In one study, CT with contrast was normal in 40 %, and LM was mistaken for parenchymal disease in 24 %, making the sensitivity less than one-third.[31]

Although a nonspecific finding, hydrocephalus seen on CT or MRI of the brain should raise the suspicion of LM.

5.3 Cerebrospinal fluid flow study

Patients with LM can have abnormal CSF flow dynamics without evidence of hydrocephalus or any other abnormality on neurologic imaging. Radioisotope ventriculography can evaluate CSF flow dynamics by measuring the distribution of the isotope throughout the subarachnoid space by gamma counter. Fifty to seventy percent of patients have evidence of CSF flow disturbance demonstrated on indium or technecium ventriculography.[22,47,53] Common sites of abnormal flow were ventricular outlet obstructions, spinal canal, and over the cortical convexities. Flow abnormality correlates with prognosis.[47,53] Patients with abnormal flow who were treated with intrathecal (IT) chemotherapy experienced significant drug toxicity and had a significantly lower survival. Patients whose flow was restored to normal after focal radiation had a better outcome. Mason et al. measured the ventricular methotrexate levels in these patients, and showed that patients with a partial spinal block who achieved a therapeutic level still had a poor prognosis.[70] They suggested that inadequate drug distribution is not the sole cause of chemotherapeutic failure; impaired flow may be an indirect measure of tumor burden within the subarachnoid space which is associated with more extensive disease and a worse prognosis.

5.4 Other diagnostic tests

The sensitivity of CT myelography for detecting LM is about 26 % [135] and similar to an MRI of the spine.[22] Small nodules seen along nerve roots can suggest the diagnosis of LM. Given the noninvasive nature of MRI, CT myelography does not have a primary role in the diagnosis of LM.

Electrophysiological tests are nonspecific but may help assist the diagnosis in some cases. For example, electroencephalography (EEG) may be able to differentiate seizure activity versus pressure waves. Nerve conduction study/electromyography may be able to differentiate root disease versus peripheral neuropathy and the finding of polyradiculopathy on EMG/NCS in a cancer patient is suggestive of LM. The diagnosis may also to be established by leptomeningeal biopsy. [9,90]

6. TREATMENT (Table 4)

Table 4. Current Treatments for Leptomeningeal Metastases

Chemotherapy		
	Intrathecal	
		Methotrexate 10-15 mg
		Cytarabine 50-100 mg
		Liposomal cytarabine 50 mg
		Thiotepa 12 mg
	Systemic	High dose Methotrexate
Radiation therapy		3000 cGy
Symptomatic		
	Ventriculoperitoneal shunt	
	Pain management	
	Anticonvulsants if a patient has seizure	

6.1 Chemotherapy (intravenous and intrathecal)

IT administration of chemotherapeutic agents is the standard of care for LM. Limited agents are commercially available, but these include methotrexate (MTX), cytosine arabinoside in the standard or liposomal preparation (Ara-C), and thiotepa. Unfortunately, these agents have limited tumoricidal activity against most solid tumors. For example, MTX and thiotepa have some tumoricidal activity against breast cancer, and thiotepa against melanoma, but none of these agents have intrinsic activity against lung cancer.[33] Nevertheless, this route has traditionally been the best way to deliver effective treatment with minimal toxicity to the entire neuraxis. Studies evaluating the efficacy of this modality have varied results. One study with breast cancer patients treated with radiation therapy and IT MTX showed an 80 % response rate with a median survival of 24 weeks and a 1-year survival rate of 25 %.[86] However, overall response rates are between 0-76 % with a median survival of 7 to 24 weeks and a 1- year survival rate of 0 to 21 %, raising the question of how efficacious these treatments are.[9, 18, 26, 37, 45, 54, 59, 86, 89, 90, 112, 123, 135 104, 139]

Administration of IT chemotherapy via Ommaya reservoir is superior to LP because it is less painful and can be done safely, even in patients with low platelets, and drug distribution throughout the subarachnoid space is superior to LP.[104] Up to 10% of chemotherapeutic agents administered through LP can escape the CSF space and end up in the epidural space, even when there is good CSF return after the placement of a needle.[67] As there is discordance between lumbar and ventricular CSF, periodic LPs to monitor response are required. As CSF volume reaches the adult level by age four and is relatively constant regardless of body habitus, a flat dose of all IT chemotherapy can be given.

MTX is an anti-metabolite and is the most widely used agent. The standard dose is 10-15 mg which reliably exceeds and remains greater than 1 uM, the therapeutic level, for at least 48 hours.[16] Initially MTX is given twice a week so therapeutic CSF levels are maintained almost continuously. There is no consensus as to how long this biweekly dose is maintained nor how long IT MTX should be continued. However, after six to eight treatments or when the CSF clears, this can be changed to weekly, and then monthly administration for at least three to six months and perhaps indefinitely depending on CSF cytology and symptoms. This type of therapy is well tolerated. MTX is reabsorbed into the bloodstream by bulk flow and transport via the choroid plexus from CSF to systemic circulation and metabolized systemically.[90] Most of the systemic toxicity of IT MTX is a result of this reabsorption; white matter changes are seen on MRI and can lead to long term neurotoxicity (primarily impaired memory). In patients treated with IT MTX, oral leucovorin (folinic acid) can be given twice a day on the day of treatment and for the following three days to prevent mucositis and myelosuppression. Leucovorin does not cross the BBB to interfere with the effect of MTX. [73]

Ara-C, a synthetic pyrimidine nucleoside analog, is an alternative agent but unfortunately is inactive in most solid tumors. Therefore, it is generally restricted to patients with hematological malignancies. A dose of 50 to 100 mg is given twice a week. Alternatively, 30 mg daily for three days can result in therapeutic concentrations for more than 72 hours. The half-life of Ara-C is very short in the serum but much longer in CSF because the enzyme cytidine deaminase is lower in the CSF. Recently, a sustained-release formulation of cytarabine (DepoCyt) for IT administration has been approved for LM from hematologic malignancies. This formulation can maintain cytotoxic concentrations of the drug for more than 14 days after a single 50 mg injection. While a survival advantage was not seen when compared to IT MTX, the time to neurological progression was slightly longer.[50] The major side effect is arachnoiditis and patients require the use of Decadron 4 mg twice a day for five days.

Thiotepa is a lipid-soluble alkylating agent with a broad spectrum of activity against solid tumors. It can be administrated as 10 mg twice weekly. It is rapidly absorbed from CSF into the systemic circulation within an hour, therefore its efficacy has been questioned. In a randomized prospective study comparing IT thiotepa to IT MTX, the overall survival was similar but patients on thiotepa had fewer toxicities.[54] Intrathecal thiotepa is myelosuppressive and should be avoided in patients with limited bone marrow reserve.[55] The use of combination IT chemotherapy has not demonstrated superiority over a single IT agent.[45, 59, 112,123]

The role of systemic IV chemotherapy is has been evaluated. Siegel et al. demonstrated that 31 patients who completed an aggressive combined modality treatment remained stable off therapy for at least six months; they also questioned the utility of IT therapy in treating these patients.[108] The authors further conducted a prospective trial comparing radiotherapy, IT chemotherapy and systemic therapy (group 1) to radiotherapy and systemic chemotherapy (group 2). The exclusion of IT chemotherapy did not change the overall response to treatment but significantly reduced treatment-related side effects.[17] Glantz et al. demonstrated that high-dose IV MTX achieved prolonged cytotoxic serum and CSF MTX concentrations, and the cytologic clearance rate and median survival were superior to the IT MTX group.[49]

There are several advantages of systemic chemotherapy over IT treatment. Most patients with LM have concomitant systemic disease and the status of systemic disease is an important prognostic factor. In these patients, it is important to treat both the systemic and leptomeningeal disease. Secondly, IT chemotherapeutic agents do not reach the core of bulky tumor as they only penetrate a few millimeters into a tumor nodule with leptomeningeal coating.[33] In bulky LM, there is neovascular formation and these new vessels do not have a BBB to prevent systemic agents from reaching the core of the tumor. This is important given that the number of IT agents is so limited. Recent reports of LM from breast and prostate cancer responding to systemic hormonal therapy and trastuzumab reinforce the principle that treatments need to be directed at the primary tumor. [7, 19, 68, 74] There are also reports of responses to systemic agents such as Xeloda for LM from breast cancer and 5-fluourouracil and gemcitabine for LM from renal carcinoma. [46, 98, 121]]

6.2 Radiation therapy

The primary role for radiation therapy is to treat symptomatic areas of bulky tumor or regions of CSF blockade; symptomatic sites, nodular disease or areas of CSF obstruction should be radiated. Response to radiation is related to the sensitivity or resistance of the primary tumor; it is palliative, but can dramatically improve signs and symptoms, especially pain.

For patients with LM, malignant cells circulate within the subarachnoid space. In order for radiation therapy to eradicate LM, the entire neuraxis must be treated. This often is not feasible: 1) The myelosuppressive effects of this treatment may prevent further systemic therapies. 2) Since the cells are circulating, it is not likely that the treatment will "kill' all the cells. Nonetheless, there are reports of patients who derived a short-lived benefit with craniospinal irradiation. [57]

Newer IT agents are actively being sought to treat LM. Chemotherapeutic agents such as mafosphamide, 4-hydroperoxycyclophosphamide, topotecan, 5-fluoro-2'deoxyuridine, interferon, busulfan and temozolomide have been investigated for IT administration.[14,15,28,43,80,100] Immunotherapy (interferon, interleukin-2, and immunotoxin), radiolabeled monoclonal antibodies targeted to specific tumor antigens, and gene therapy introducing "suicide" genes are some of the novel approaches currently under investigation.[13,30,58,76,134]

Patients with LM often develop communicating hydrocephalus. Placement of ventriculoperitoneal (VP) shunt can give marked and immediate relief of symptoms and although palliative, may be the most effective intervention in the treatment of LM. Even without a radiographically evident hydrocephalus on neuroimaging, patients can still have increased ICP and symptoms can be relieved by this procedure. There is a theoretical concern of tumor seeding the peritoneal cavity, but this concern is probably clinically irrelevant. [90] IT chemotherapy after shunting is a difficult management issue and may increase the reliance on systemic therapy. It is possible to place a VP shunt with an "on-off" valve and turn the shunt off for several hours after IT administration of chemotherapy.
Patients must be able to tolerate having the shunt off for a few hours. Unfortunately, the drug may not circulate as effectively as the CSF flow

dynamics are significantly altered in these patients. Additionally, transependymal resorption of chemotherapeutic agents may increase the neurotoxicity of IT chemotherapies. Therefore, if IT chemotherapy is considered, LP may be an alternative route allowing the drug to enter and contact the spinal leptomeninges, the basal cisterns, and finally the ventricles and exit via the shunt.[2]

6.3 Complications

Patients with LM are subjected to the general side effects of radiation therapy and systemic chemotherapy specific to each agent. Complications from Ommaya placement occur in 2-9 % of patients and include perioperative complications, inappropriate placement, migration of the catheter tip from the ventricle into the adjacent brain tissue, infections or intracranial hemorrhage.[25, 84, 101, 124] To ensure proper placement, a CT scan should be done prior to placing the Ommaya reservoir. About 5 % of reservoirs become infected at some time during therapy. The most common organisms are Staphylococcus epidermis and Propionibacterium acnes.[25, 124] Most of the infections are asymptomatic, but at times patients develop symptoms of meningitis. IV or intra-Ommaya antibiotics can effectively sterilize the subarachnoid space in most cases.[25, 101, 116] If the infection cannot be cleared with medical management, the reservoir must be removed. A new reservoir can be inserted once the infection resolves and treatment can continue.[116, 124]

Side effects related to injection of chemotherapy are rare. Up to 5% of patients will develop a chemical meningitis following IT chemotherapy; the risk may be higher with DepoCyt therapy where all patients require corticosteroids for 72 hours after treatment. Seizures and unexplained death have been reported as acute side effects.[84, 125] Delayed side effects include white matter necrosis around the catheter tract, introduction of infection from aseptic technique, leukoencephalopathy, and myelosuppression. Leukoencephalopathy occurs in 3–5% of cases and is associated with a previous history of radiation and MTX, and reduced clearance secondary to CSF flow abnormality.[25, 84, 86, 101] Mild memory problems and gait disturbance, even without evident white matter changes, are common and may respond to placement of a VP shunt.[119]

7. PROGNOSIS

The prognosis of LM from solid tumor remains poor. The median survival is four to six weeks without treatment. Treatment can stabilize the neurological symptoms and prolong survival for a few months but less than

10% of patients are alive after one year. Breast cancer has the best prognosis; about 15% of patients survive more than a year.[120,75] Prognosis remains poor in patients with lung cancer and melanoma.[26] In these patients, some clinicians question the usefulness of vigorous treatment and favor palliative care once the diagnosis is made. There are some conflicting data in regards to prognostic factors, but in general, patients with breast cancer (especially if progesterone positive), a better performance status (Karnofsky performance scale > 60), controlled systemic cancer, absence of bulky disease, normal CSF protein, absence of cerebral involvement and a chemosensitive primary, benefit the most from aggressive treatment.[9, 18, 23, 24, 34, 55, 89]

8. CLINICAL GUIDELINES

When a patient with solid tumor presents with multiple neurological symptoms or signs, LM needs to be ruled out. In addition, LM should be considered in a patient with incidental finding of hydrocephalus. MRI with and without gadolinium of the involved area is the test of choice; if positive, the whole neuro-axis should be evaluated. If MRI is negative, the CSF needs to be examined. Repeat examination of CSF, including cisternal puncture may be necessary to make the diagnosis of LM. Occasionally, treatment decisions are based on clinical findings despite a negative work up.

After the diagnosis of LM is established, a VP shunt should be placed if hydrocephalus is present. Radiation therapy is then given to symptomatic sites, nodular lesions, or areas of CSF blockage. If the patient has breast cancer, and good prognostic factors, an Ommaya device can be placed and IT MTX can be considered. Alternatively, it is reasonable to treat the LM and concomitant systemic disease with systemic chemotherapy; agents used should have activity against the primary tumor with CSF penetration. If the patient has a poor prognosis, symptomatic therapy and palliative care should be the focus.

REFERENCES

1. Eberth CJ. Zur Entwicklung des Epitheliomas (Cholesteatomas) dur Pia under der Lungs. Virchow's Arch 1870; 49:51-63.
2. Posner, JB. "Leptomeningeal Metastases." In *Neurological complication of cancer*, Posner JB, Philadelphia, PA: F.A. Davis Co., 1995.
3. Grossman SA, Krabak MJ. Leptomeningeal carcinomatosis. Cancer Treat Rev 1999; 25:103-1979.
4. DeAngelis LM. Current diagnosis and treatment of leptomeningeal metastasis. J Neurooncol 1998; 38:245-52.

5. Freilich RJ, Seidman AD, DeAngelis LM. Central nervous system progression of metastatic breast cancer in patients treated with paclitaxel. Cancer 1995; 76:232-6.
6. Bishop JR Jr, Moul JW, Maldonado L, McLeod DG. Transitional cell carcinomatous meningitis after M-VAC (methotrexate, vinblastine, doxorubicin, and cisplatin) chemotherapy. Urology 1990; 36:373-7.
7. Posner JB, Chernik NL. Intracranial metastasis from systemic cancer. Adv Neurol 1978; 19:575-587.
8. Glass JP, Melamed M, Chernik NL, Posner JB. Malignant cells in cerebrospinal fluid (CSF): The meaning of a positive cytology. Neurology 1979; 29:1369-1375.
9. Olson ME, Chernik NL, Posner JB. Infiltration of the leptomeninges by systemic cancer. A clinical and pathologic study. Arch Neurol 1974; 30:122-37.
10. Wasserstrom WR, Glass JP, Posner JB. Diagnosis and treatment of leptomeningeal metastases from solid tumors: experience with 90 patients. Cancer 1982; 49:759-72.
11. Balm M, Hammack J. Leptomeningeal carcinomatosis. Presenting features and prognostic factors. Arch Neurol 1996; 53:626-32.
12. Aisner J, Aisner SC, Ostrow S, Govindan S, Mummert K, Wiernik P. Meningeal carcinomatosis from small cell carcinoma of the lung. Consequence of improved survival. Acta Cytol 1979; 23:292-9.
13. Aroney RS, Dalley DN, Chan WK, Bell DR, Levi JA. Meningeal carcinomatosis in small cell carcinoma of the lung. Am J Med 1981; 71:26-32.
14. Balducci L, Little DD, Khansur T, Steinberg MH. Carcinomatous meningitis in small cell lung cancer. Am J Med Sci 1984; 287:31-3.
15. Rosen ST, Aisner J, Makuch RW, et al. Carcinomatous leptomeningitis in small cell lung cancer: a clinicopathologic review of the National Cancer Institute experience. Medicine (Baltimore). 1982; 61:45-53.
16. Auperin A, Arriagada R, Pignon JP, et al. RT for Small cell. Prophylactic cranial irradiation for patients with small-cell lung cancer in complete remission. Prophylactic Cranial Irradiation Overview Collaborative Group. N Engl J Med 1999; 341:476-84.
17. Jayson GC, Howell A, Harris M, Morgenstern G, Chang J, Ryder WD. Carcinomatous meningitis in patients with breast cancer. An aggressive disease variant. Cancer 1994; 74:3135-41.
18. Tsukada Y, Fouad A, Pickren JW, Lane WW. Central nervous system metastasis from breast carcinoma. Autopsy study. Cancer 1983; 52:2349-54.
19. Yap HY, Yap BS, Tashima CK, DiStefano A, Blumenschein GR. Meningeal carcinomatosis in breast cancer. Cancer 1978; 42:283-6.
20. De la Monte SM, Hutchins GM, Moore GW. Estrogen and progesterone receptors in prediction of metastatic behavior of breast carcinoma. Am J Med 1984; 76:11-7.
21. Amer MH, Al-Sarraf M, Baker LH, Vaitkevicius VK. Malignant melanoma and central nervous system metastases: incidence, diagnosis, treatment and survival. Cancer 1978; 42:660-8.
22. Crino PB, Sater RA, Sperling M, Katsetos CD. Renal cell carcinomatous meningitis: pathologic and immunohistochemical features. Neurology 1995; 45:189-91.
23. Mencel PJ, DeAngelis LM, Motzer RJ. Hormonal ablation as effective therapy for carcinomatous meningitis from prostatic carcinoma. Cancer 1994; 73:1892-4.
24. Strady C, Ricciarelli A, Nasca S, Liautaud-Roger F, Coninx P. Carcinomatous meningitis and solid tumours. Oncol Rep 2000; 7:203-7.
25. Fisher MA, Weiss RB. Carcinomatous meningitis in gastrointestinal malignancies. South Med J 1979; 72:930-2.
26. Mayer RJ, Berkowitz RS, Griffiths CT. Central nervous system involvement by ovarian carcinoma: a complication of prolonged survival with metastatic disease. Cancer 1978;

41:776-83.
27. Vadmal MS, Brones C, Farmer PM. Recurrent adenocarcinoma of the fallopian tube presenting as leptomeningeal carcinomatosis. Ann Clin Lab Sci 1996; 26:119-21.
28. Aboulafia DM, Taylor LP, Crane RD, Yon JL, Rudolph RH. Carcinomatous meningitis complicating cervical cancer: a clinicopathologic study and literature review. Gynecol Oncol 1996; 60:313-8.
29. Redman BG, Tapazoglou E, Al-Sarraf M. Meningeal carcinomatosis in head and neck cancer. Report of six cases and review of the literature. Cancer 1986; 58:2656-61.
30. Barnard RO, Parsons M. Carcinoma of the thyroid with leptomeningeal dissemination following the treatment of a toxic goitre with 131-I and methyl thiouracil. Case with a co-existing intracranial dermoid. J Neurol Sci 1969; 8:299-306.
31. Kramer K, Kushner B, Heller G, Cheung NK. Neuroblastoma metastatic to the central nervous system. The Memorial Sloan-Kettering Cancer Center Experience and A Literature Review. Cancer 2001; 91:1510-9.
32. Eggers SD, Salomao DR, Dinapoli RP, Vernino S. Paraneoplastic and metastatic neurologic complications of Merkel cell carcinoma. Mayo Clin Proc 2001; 76:327-30.
33. Nagourney RA, Hedaya R, Linnoila M, Schein PS. Carcinoid carcinomatous meningitis. Ann Intern Med 1985; 102:779-82.
34. Kline RM, Oseas RS, Jolley SG, et al. Leptomeningeal metastasis from a paraspinal rhabdomyosarcoma with a der(13)t(1;13)(q23;q32) in a 14-month-old boy. Cancer Genet Cytogenet 1997; 98:97-101.
35. Begemann M, Rosenblum MK, Loh J, et al. Leptomeningeal Metastases from recurrent squamous cell cancer of the skin. J Neurooncol 2003; 63: 295-298.
36. Thompson SR, Veness MJ, Morgan GJ, Shannon J, Kenech JG. Leptomeningeal carcinomatosis from squamous cell carcinoma of the supraglottic larynx. Australas Radiol 2003; 47: 325-330.
37. Zhu JJ, Padillo O, Duff J, Hsi BL, Fletcher JA, Querfurth H. Cavernous sinus and leptomeningeal metastases arising from a squamous cell carcinoma of the face: case report. Neurosurgery 2004; 54: 492-8.
38. Kokkoris CP. Leptomeningeal carcinomatosis. How does cancer reach the pia-arachnoid? Cancer 1983; 51:154-60.
39. Price RA and Johnson WW. The central nervous system in childhood leukemia. I. The arachnoid. Cancer 1973; 58:520-533.
40. Norris LK, Grossman SA, Olivi A. Neoplastic meningitis following surgical resection of isolated cerebellar metastasis: a potentially preventable complication. J Neurooncol 1997; 32:215-23.
41. van der Ree TC, Dippel DW, Avezaat CJ, Sillevis Smitt PA, Vecht CJ, van den Bent MJ. Leptomeningeal metastasis after surgical resection of brain metastases. J Neurol Neurosurg Psychiatry 1999; 66:225-7.
42. Klein P, Haley EC, Wooten GF, VandenBerg SR. Focal cerebral infarctions associated with perivascular tumor infiltrates in carcinomatous leptomeningeal metastases. Arch Neurol 1989; 46:1149- 52.
43. Siegal T, Mildworf B, Stein D, Melamed E. Leptomeningeal metastases: reduction in regional cerebral blood flow and cognitive impairment. Ann Neurol 1985; 17:100-2.
44. Kaplan JG, DeSouza TG, Farkash A, et al. Leptomeningeal metastases: comparison of clinical features and laboratory data of solid tumors, lymphomas and leukemias. J Neurooncol 1990; 9:225-9.
45. van Oostenbrugge RJ, Hopman AH, Arends JW, Ramaekers FC, Twijnstra A. The value of interphase cytogenetics in cytology for the diagnosis of leptomeningeal metastases. Neurology 1998; 51:906-8.

46. Wolfgang G, Marcus D, Ulrike S. LC: clinical syndrome in different primaries. J Neurooncol 1998; 38:103-10.

47. Tham LC, Millward MJ, Lind MJ, Cantwell BM. Metastatic breast cancer presenting with diabetes insipidus. Acta Oncol 1992; 31:679-80.

48. Oster JR, Perez GO, Larios O, Emery WE, Bourgoignie JJ. Cerebral salt wasting in a man with carcinomatous meningitis. Arch Intern Med 1983; 143:2187-8.

49. Broderick JP, Cascino TL. Nonconvulsive status epilepticus in a patient with leptomeningeal cancer. Mayo Clin Proc. 1987; 62:835-7.

50. Marcus FS, Dandolos EM, Friedman MA. Meningeal carcinomatosis in breast cancer presenting as central hypoventilation: a case report with a brief review of the literature. Cancer 1981; 47:982-4.

51. Weitzner MA, Olofsson SM, Forman AD. Patients with malignant meningitis presenting with neuropsychiatric manifestations. Cancer 1995; 76:1804-8.

52. Sozzi G, Marotta P, Piatti L. Vagoglossopharyngeal neuralgia with syncope in the course of carcinomatous meningitis. Ital J Neurol Sci 1987; 8:271-5.

53. Guarino M, Stracciari A, Cirignotta F, D'Alessandro R, Pazzaglia P. Neoplastic meningitis presenting with ophthalmoplegia, ataxia, and areflexia (Miller-Fisher syndrome) Arch Neurol 1995; 52:443-4.

54. Glantz MJ, Cole BF, Glantz LK, et al. Cerebrospinal fluid cytology in patients with cancer: minimizing false-negative results. Cancer 1998; 82:733-9.

55. Chamberlain MC, Kormanik PA, Glantz MJ. A comparison between ventricular and lumbar cerebrospinal fluid cytology in adult patients with leptomeningeal metastases. J Neuro-Oncol 2001; 3:42-5.

56. Rogers LR, Duchesneau PM, Nunez C, et al. Comparison of cisternal and lumbar CSF examination in leptomeningeal metastasis. Neurology 1992; 42:1239-41.

57. Raizer JJ, DeAngelis LM. Cerebral sinus thrombosis diagnosed by MRI and MR venography in cancer patients. Neurology 2000; 54:1222-6.

58. van Zanten AP, Twijnstra A, Ongerboer de Visser BW, van Heerde P, Hart AA, Nooyen WJ. Cerebrospinal fluid tumour markers in patients treated for meningeal malignancy. J Neurol Neurosurg Psychiatry 1991; 54:119-23.

59. Schold SC, Wasserstrom WR, Fleisher M, Schwartz MK, Posner JB. Cerebrospinal fluid biochemical markers of central nervous system metastases. Ann Neurol 1980; 8:597-604.

60. Lampl Y, Paniri Y, Eshel Y, Sarova-Pinchas I. Alkaline phosphatase level in CSF in various brain tumors and pulmonary carcinomatous meningitis. J Neurooncol 1990; 9:35-40.

61. Sato Y, Ohta Y, Kaji M, Oizumi K, Kaji M. Carbohydrate antigen 19-9 in cerebrospinal fluid and within malignant cells in a case of leptomeningeal carcinomatosis. J Neurol Neurosurg Psychiatry 1998; 65:402-3.

62. Castro MP, McDonald TJ, Qualman SJ, Odorisio TM. Cerebrospinal fluid gastrin releasing peptide in the diagnosis of leptomeningeal metastases from small cell carcinoma. Cancer 2001; 91:2122-6.

63. Fleisher M, Wasserstrom WR, Schold SC, Schwartz MK, Posner JB. Lactic dehydrogenase isoenzymes in the cerebrospinal fluid of patients with systemic cancer. Cancer 1981 Jun; 47:2654-9.

64. Twijnstra A, van Zanten AP, Nooyen WJ, Hart AA, Ongerboer de Visser BW. Cerebrospinal fluid beta 2-microglobulin: a study in controls and patients with metastatic and non-metastatic neurological diseases. Eur J Cancer Clin Oncol 1986; 22:387-91.

65. Twijnstra A, van Zanten AP, Nooyen WJ, Ongerboer de Visser BW. Sensitivity and specificity of single and combined tumour markers in the diagnoses of leptomeningeal metastases from breast cancer. J Neurol Neurosurg Psychiatry 1986: 49; 1246-50.

66. Siegal T, Ovadia H, Yatsiv I, Abramsky O. CSF myelin basic protein levels in

leptomeningeal metastases. Relationship to disease activity. J Neurol Sci 1987; 78:165-73.
67. Zandman-Goddard G, Matzner Y, Konijn AM, Hershko C. Cerebrospinal fluid ferritin in malignant CNS involvement. Cancer 1986; 58:1346-9.
68. Moseley RP, Oge K, Shafqat S, et al. HMFG1 antigen: a new marker for carcinomatous meningitis. Int J Cancer 1989; 44:440-4.
69. Nakamura S, Nagano I, Yoshioka M, et al. Immunocytochemical detection of tumor necrosis factor-alpha in infiltrating tumor cells in the cerebrospinal fluid from five patients with leptomeningeal carcinomatosis. Acta Neurol Scand 1995; 91:137-40.
70. Stockhammer G, Poewe W, Burgstaller S, et al. Vascular endothelial growth factor in CSF: a biological marker for carcinomatous meningitis. Neurology 2000;54:1670-6.
71. Friedberg MH, Glantz MJ, Klempner MS, Cole BF, Perides G. Specific matrix metallproteinase profiles in the cerebrospinal fluid correlated with the presence of malignant astrocytoma, brain metastases, and carcinomatous meningitis. Cancer 1998; 82: 923-930.
72. Nagai A, Terashima M, Harada T, et al. Cathepsin B and H activities and cystatin C concentrations in cerebrospinal fluid from patients with leptomeningeal metastasis. Clin Chim Acta 2003; 329: 53-60.
73. Cibas ES, Malkin MG, Posner JB, Melamed MR. Detection of DNA abnormalities by flow cytometry in cells from cerebrospinal fluid. Am J Clin Pathol 1987 88:570-7.
74. Fujita J, Ueda Y, Bandoh S, Namihira H, Ishii T, Takahara J. A case of leptomeningeal metastasis from lung adenocarcinoma diagnosed by reverse transcriptase-polymerase chain reaction for carcinoembryonic antigen. Lung Cancer 1998; 22:153-6.
75. Swinkels DW, de Kok JB, Hanselaar A, Lamers K, Boerman RH. Early detection of leptomeningeal metastasis by PCR examination of tumor-derived K-ras DNA in cerebrospinal fluid. Clin Chem 2000; 46:132-3.
76. van Oostenbrugge RJ, Hopman AH, Arends JW, Ramaekers FC, Twijnstra A. Treatment of leptomeningeal metastases evaluated by interphase cytogenetics. J Clin Oncol 2000: 18; 2053-8.
77. Freilich RJ, Krol G, DeAngelis LM. Neuroimaging and cerebrospinal fluid cytology in the diagnosis of leptomeningeal metastasis. Ann Neurol 1995; 38:51-7.
78. Collie DA, Brush JP, Lammie GA, et al. Imaging features of leptomeningeal metastases. Clin Radiol 1999; 54:765-71.
79. Straathof CS, de Bruin HG, Dippel DW, Vecht CJ. The diagnostic accuracy of magnetic resonance imaging and cerebrospinal fluid cytology in leptomeningeal metastasis. J Neurol. 1999; 246:810-4.
80. River Y, Schwartz A, Gomori JM, Soffer D, Siegal T. Clinical significance of diffuse dural enhancement detected by magnetic resonance imaging. J Neurosurg 1996; 85:777-83.
81. Abrey LE, Rosenblum MK, DeAngelis LM. Sarcoidosis of the cauda equina mimicking leptomeningeal malignancy. J Neurooncol 1998; 39:261-5
82. Gorson KC, Ropper AH, Muriello MA, Blair R. Prospective evaluation of MRI lumbosacral nerve root enhancement in acute Guillain-Barré syndrome. Neurology 1996; 47:813-7.
83. Singh SK, Agris JM, Leeds NE, Ginsberg LE. Intracranial leptomeningeal metastases: comparison of depiction at FLAIR and contrast-enhanced MR imaging. Radiology 2000; 217:50-3.
84. Mathews VP, Caldemeyer KS, Lowe MJ, Greenspan SL, Weber DM, Ulmer JL. Brain: gadolinium-enhanced fast fluid-attenuated inversion-recovery MR imaging. Radiology 1999; 211:257-63.
85. Singh SK, Leeds, NE, Ginsberg LE. MR imaging of leptomeningeal metastases: Comparison of three sequences. Am J Neuroradiol 2002; 23: 817-821.
86. Glantz MJ, Hall WA, Cole BF, et al. Diagnosis, management, and survival of patients

with leptomeningeal cancer based on cerebrospinal fluid-flow status. Cancer 1995; 75:2919-31.
87. Chamberlain MC, Kormanik PA. Prognostic significance of 111indium-DTPA CSF flow studies in leptomeningeal metastases. Neurology 1996; 46:1674-7.
88. Grossman SA, Trump DL, Chen DC, Thompson G, Camargo EE. Cerebrospinal fluid flow abnormalities in patients with neoplastic meningitis. An evaluation using 111indium-DTPA ventriculography. Am J Med 1982; 73:641-7.
89. Mason WP, Yeh SD, DeAngelis LM. 111Indium-diethylenetriamine pentaacetic acid cerebrospinal fluid flow studies predict distribution of intrathecally administered chemotherapy and outcome in patients with leptomeningeal metastases. Neurology 1998; 50:438-44.
90. Chamberlain MC. Comparative spine imaging in leptomeningeal metastases. J Neurooncol. 1995; 23:233-8.
91. Ongerboer de Visser BW, Somers R, Nooyen WH, van Heerde P, Hart AA, McVie JG. Intraventricular methotrexate therapy of leptomeningeal metastasis from breast carcinoma. Neurology 1983; 33:1565-72.
92. Boogerd W, Hart AA, van der Sande JJ, Engelsman E. Meningeal carcinomatosis in breast cancer. Prognostic factors and influence of treatment. Cancer 1991; 67:1685-95.
93. Chamberlain MC, Kormanik P. Carcinoma meningitis secondary to non-small cell lung cancer: combined modality therapy. Arch Neurol 1998; 55:506-12.
94. Esteva FJ, Soh LT, Holmes FA, et al. Phase II trial and pharmacokinetic evaluation of cytosine arabinoside for leptomeningeal metastases from breast cancer. Cancer Chemother Pharmacol 2000; 46:382-6.
95. Giannone L, Greco FA, Hainsworth JD. Combination intraventricular chemotherapy for meningeal neoplasia. J Clin Oncol 1986; 4:68-73.
96. Grossman SA, Finkelstein DM, Ruckdeschel JC, Trump DL, Moynihan T, Ettinger DS. Randomized prospective comparison of intraventricular methotrexate and thiotepa in patients with previously untreated neoplastic meningitis. Eastern Cooperative Oncology Group. J Clin Oncol 1993; 11:561-9.
97. Hitchins RN, Bell DR, Woods RL, Levi JA. A prospective randomized trial of single-agent versus combination chemotherapy in meningeal carcinomatosis. J Clin Oncol 1987; 5:1655-62.
98. Pfeffer MR, Wygoda M, Siegal T. Leptomeningeal metastases--treatment results in 98 consecutive patients. Isr J Med Sci 1988; 24:611-8.
99. Stewart DJ, Maroun JA, Hugenholtz H, et al. Combined intra Ommaya methotrexate, cytosine arabinoside, hydrocortisone and thio-TEPA for meningeal involvement by malignancies. J Neurooncol 1987; 5:315-22.
100. Trump DL, Grossman SA, Thompson G, Murray K, Wharam M. Treatment of neoplastic meningitis with intraventricular thiotepa and methotrexate. Cancer Treat Rep 1982; 66:1549-51.
101. Shapiro WR, Posner JB, Ushio Y, Chemik NL, Young DF. Treatment of meningeal neoplasms. Cancer Treat Rep 1977; 61:733-43.
102. Yap HY, Yap BS, Rasmussen S, Levens ME, Hortobagyi GN, Blumenschein GR. Treatment for meningeal carcinomatosis in breast cancer. Cancer 1982; 50:219-22.
103. Shapiro WR, Young DF, Mehta BM. Methotrexate: distribution in cerebrospinal fluid after intravenous, ventricular and lumbar injections. N Engl J Med 1975; 93:161-6.
104. Larson SM, Schall GL, Di Chiro G. The influence of previous lumbar puncture and pneumoencephalography on the incidence of unsuccessful radioisotope cisternography. J Nucl Med 1971; 2:555-7.
105. Bleyer WA, Coccia PF, Sather HN, et al. Reduction in central nervous system leukemia

with a pharmacokinetically derived intrathecal methotrexate dosage regimen. J Clin Oncol 1983; 1:317-25.

106. Mehta BM, Glass JP, Shapiro WR. Serum and cerebrospinal fluid distribution of 5-methyltetrahydrofolate after intravenous calcium leucovorin and intra-Ommaya methotrexate administration in patients with meningeal carcinomatosis. Cancer Res 1983; 43:435-8.

107. Glantz MJ, Jaeckle KA, Chamberlain MC, et al. A randomized controlled trial comparing intrathecal sustained-release cytarabine (DepoCyt) to intrathecal methotrexate in patients with neoplastic meningitis from solid tumors. Clin Cancer Res 1999; 5:3394-402.

108. Siegal T, Lossos A, Pfeffer MR. Leptomeningeal metastases: analysis of 31 patients with sustained off-therapy response following combined-modality therapy. Neurology 1994; 44:1463-9.

109. Bokstein F, Lossos A, Siegal T. Leptomeningeal metastases from solid tumors: a comparison of two prospective series treated with and without intra-cerebrospinal fluid chemotherapy. Cancer 1998; 82:1756-63.

110. Glantz MJ, Cole BF, Recht L, et al. High-dose intravenous methotrexate for patients with nonleukemic leptomeningeal cancer: is intrathecal chemotherapy necessary? J Clin Oncol 1998; 16:1561-7.

111. Baculi RH, Suki S, Nisbett J, Leeds N, Groves M. Meningeal carcinomatosis from breast carcinoma responsive to trastuzumab. J Clin Oncol 2001; 19:3297-8.

112. Boogerd W, Dorresteijn LD, van Der Sande JJ, de Gast GC, Bruning PF. Response of leptomeningeal metastases from breast cancer to hormonal therapy. Neurology 2000; 55:117-9.

113. Laufman LR, Forsthoefel KF. Use of intrathecal trastuzumab in a patient with carcinomatous meningitis. Clin Breast Cancer 2001; 2: 235.

114. Giglio P, Tremont-Lukats IW, Groves MD. Response of neoplastic meningitis from solid tumors to oral capecitabine. J Neuro-Oncol 2003; 65:167-72

115. Roger LR, Remer SE, Tejwani S. Durable response of breast cancer leptomeningeal metastases to capecitabine monotherapy. Neuro-Oncol 2004; 6: 63-4.

116. Tippin DB, Reeves W, Vogelzang NJ. Diagnosis and treatment of leptomeningeal metastases in a patient with renal carcinoma responding to 5-flourouracil and gemcitabine. J Urol 1999; 162:'155-6.

117. Hermann B, Hultenschmidt B, Sautter-Bihl ML. Radiotherapy of the neuro-axis for palliative treatment of leptomeningeal carcinomatosis. Strahlenther Onkol 2001; 177: 195-9.

118. Blaney SM, Poplack DG. New cytotoxic drugs for intrathecal administration. J Neurooncol 1998; 38:219-23.

119. Blaney SM, Heidman R, Berg S, et al. Phase I clinical trail of intrathecal topotecan in patients with neoplastic meningitis. J Clin Oncol 2003; 21: 143-7.

120. Chamberlain MC. A phase II trial of intra-cerebrospinal fluid alpha interferon in the treatment of neoplastic meningitis. Cancer 2002; 94: 2675-80.

121. Friedman HS. Temozolomide in early stages of newly diagnosed malignant glioma and neoplastic meningitis. Semin Oncol 2000; 27(3 Suppl 6): 35-40.

122. Nakagawa H, Yamada M, Fukushima M, Ikenaka K. Intrathecal 5-fluoro-2'-deoxyuridine (FdUrd) for the treatment of solid tumor neoplastic meningitis: an in vivo study. Cancer Chemother Pharmacol 1999; 43:247-56.

123. Sampson JH, Archer GE, Villavicencio AT, et al. Treatment of neoplastic meningitis with intrathecal temozolomide. Clin Cancer Res 1999; 5:1183-8.

124. Quinn JA, Glantz M, Petros W, et al. Phase I trial of spartaject busulfan for patients with neoplastic meningitis. Proceedings ASCO 2002, Abstract 318.

125. Bigner DD, Brown M, Coleman RE, et al. Phase I studies of treatment of malignant gliomas and neoplastic meningitis with 131I-radiolabeled monoclonal antibodies anti-tenascin

81C6 and anti-chondroitin proteoglycan sulfate Mel-14 F (ab') 2--a preliminary report. J Neurooncol 1995; 24: 109-22.

126. Coakham HB, Kemshead JT. Treatment of neoplastic meningitis by targeted radiation using (131)I-radiolabelled monoclonal antibodies. Results of responses and long term follow-up in 40 patients. J Neurooncol 1998; 38:225-32.

127. Herrlinger U, Weller M, Schabet M. New aspects of immunotherapy of leptomeningeal metastasis. J Neurooncol 1998; 38:233-9.

128. Moseley RP, Davies AG, Richardson RB, et al. Intrathecal administration of I131 radiolabeled monoclonal antibody as a treatment from neoplastic meningitis. Br J Cancer 1990; 62: 673-42.

129. Vrionis FD. Gene therapy of neoplastic meningosis. J Neurooncol 1998; 38:241-4.

130. Chamberlain MC, Kormanik PA, Barba D. Complications associated with intraventricular chemotherapy in patients with leptomeningeal metastases. J Neurosurg 1997; 87:694-9.

131. Obbens EA, Leavens ME, Beal JW, Lee YY. Ommaya reservoirs in 387 cancer patients: a 15-year experience. Neurology 1985; 35:1274-8.

132. Sandberg DI, Bilsky MH, Souweidane MM, Bzdil J, Gutin PH. Ommaya reservoirs for the treatment of leptomeningeal metastases. Neurosurgery 2000; 47:49-54.

133. Trump DL, Grossman SA, Thompson G, Murray K. CSF infections complicating the management of neoplastic meningitis. Clinical features and results of therapy. Arch Intern Med 1982; 142:583-6.

134. Sutherland GE, Palitang EG, Marr JJ, Luedke SL. Sterilization of Ommaya reservoir by instillation of vancomycin. Am J Med 1981; 71:1068-70.

135. ten Hoeve RF, Twijnstra A. A lethal neurotoxic reaction after intraventricular methotrexate administration. Cancer 1988; 62:2111-3.

136. Thiessen B, DeAngelis LM. Hydrocephalus in radiation leukoencephalopathy: results of ventriculoperitoneal shunting. Arch Neurol 1998; 55:705-10.

137. Moots PL, Harrison MB, Vandenberg SR. Prolonged survival in carcinomatous meningitis associated with breast cancer. South Med J 1995; 88:357-62.

138. Chamberlain MC, Kormanik PA. Prognostic significance of coexistent bulky metastatic central nervous system disease in patients with leptomeningeal metastases. Arch Neurol 1997; 54:1364-8.

139. Chamberlain MC, Kormanik PR. Carcinomatous meningitis secondary to breast cancer: predictors of response to combined modality therapy. J Neurooncol 1997; 35:55-64.

Chapter 4

LEPTOMENINGEAL METASTASES FROM LEUKEMIAS AND LYMPHOMAS

Craig P. Nolan, M.D., Lauren E. Abrey, M.D.
Department of Neurology, Memorial Sloan-Kettering Cancer Center, 12745 York Avenue, New York, NY 10021

Abstract: Leptomeningeal dissemination of lymphoma and leukemia differs from that of solid tumors in a number of clinically important aspects. Specific histologic variants of lymphoma and leukemia have such a high incidence of cerebrospinal fluid (CSF) dissemination that assessing CSF cytology at diagnosis is crucial and prophylactic therapy of the CSF compartment is required. Furthermore, while the overall prognosis for patients with leptomeningeal metastases from leukemia and lymphoma is similar to solid tumors, selected patients have excellent response to therapy and attain durable remission. Therefore, aggressive treatment is warranted.

Key words: Leukemia; lymphoma; acute lymphoblastic leukemia; AIDS; prophylaxis.

1. INTRODUCTION

While leptomeningeal metastases (LM) are estimated to occur in approximately 5% of all patients with cancer, the incidence of LM from leukemias and lymphomas may be underestimated in most series.[1] This may be due to the greater prevalence of solid tumors compared to hematologic malignancies. Also, in contrast to patients with solid tumors, those with LM from leukemias and lymphomas often present without evidence of systemic disease or during periods of remission. In a review of 63 cases, Kaplan *et al.* found that LM from solid tumors occurred in patients with advanced systemic disease in 90% of the cases, as compared to patients with leukemia and lymphoma whose LM occurred without systemic disease in 18 and 13%, respectively, or during remission in 35 and 27%, respectively.[2]

LM may also be the initial presentation of leukemia or lymphoma. LM from leukemias and lymphomas typically have a different clinical presentation than LM from solid tumors. Although the clinical presentation is extremely variable, LM from hematologic malignancies present with a greater incidence of cranial nerve palsies. In a study of 45 patients with LM, van Oostenbrugge found that patients with solid tumor LM presented mostly with spinal or radicular symptoms (53%) whereas patients with hematologic LM presented more frequently with cranial nerve dysfunction (53%); 67% displayed multifocal neurologic symptoms.[3]

The diagnostic approach to LM from leukemias and lymphomas is not significantly different from that of solid tumors and includes both radiographic imaging of the neuroaxis and cerebrospinal fluid (CSF) examination. Therapeutic options are also similar and include cranial-spinal irradiation, systemic chemotherapy, and intrathecal (IT) chemotherapy. Prognosis may be better than for solid tumor patients. Prophylactic treatment using intrathecal chemotherapy with or without cranial radiation may be beneficial in extending the survival in certain patients with hematologic malignancies.

Staging Lumbar Puncture Recommended

- Any acute leukemia
- Pediatric non-Hodgkin's lymphoma
- Testicular lymphoma
- Lymphoma involving the orbit or paranasal sinuses
- High grade non-Hodgkin's lymphoma
  - lymphoblastic lymphoma
  - diffuse large B-cell lymphoma

CNS Prophylaxis* Recommended

- Acute Lymphocytic Leukemia
- Burkitt's lymphoma
- Diffuse large B-cell lymphoma (International prognostic index grade IV)
- Lymphoma of the orbit or paranasal sinuses
- Testicular lymphoma (controversial)
- T-cell lymphoma (pediatrics)

* intrathecal methotrexate with or without cranial radiation

2. LYMPHOMA

The malignant lymphomas are neoplastic transformations of cells within the lymphatic system. Hodgkin's and non-Hodgkin's lymphoma (NHL) have distinct biological and clinical behaviors. Although both malignancies are sensitive to radiation therapy and chemotherapy, NHL is a more aggressive cancer with a cure rate less than 25%.[4]

Whereas LM are rarely reported in Hodgkin's lymphoma.[5,6] they occur in 5-10% of NHL patients. The occurrence of central nervous system (CNS) disease in NHL usually predicts a poor clinical outcome. This section will focus upon the incidence and risk factors for LM in NHL as well as the clinical presentation, treatment, and outcome of the disease.

2.1 Incidence

The incidence of NHL has risen over the past several decades and currently accounts for approximately 50% of all cases of leukemias and lymphomas.[4] The incidence of CNS involvement in NHL, as reported in the literature, is variable and closely associated with certain clinical risk factors for the disease (see below). Patients with NHL are not at uniform risk of developing CNS disease. CNS disease from NHL more often involves the leptomeninges than the parenchyma. In a review of a multiple series of NHL and CNS disease, Bishop *et al.* reported that CNS disease occurs in the leptomeninges and dura in 65% of cases, in the brain parenchyma in 26%, and in both the leptomeninges and parenchyma in 9% (see Table 1).[7]

Table 1. Sites of CNS Involvement in Large-Cell Lymphoma

		Leptomeningeal		Parenchymal		Both sites	
Study	Total No. of Pts.	No. of Pts.(%)		No. of Pts.	(%)	No. of Pts.	(%)
Bollen 1997 65	21	(32)	27	(42)	17	(26)	
Keldsen 1996	27	9	(33)	15	(56)	3	(11)
Bashir 1991 14	11	(79)	3	(21)	0	(0)	
Wolf 1985 44	23	(52)	20	(45)	1	(2)	
Johnson 1984	29	23	(79)	3	(10)	3	(10)
Levitt 1980 52	44	(85)	8	(15)	0	(0)	
Herman 1979	50	40	(80)	9	(18)	1	(2)
Litam 1979 31	26	(84)	4	(13)	1	(3)	
Young 1979 20	16	(80)	2	(10)	2	(10)	
Law 1975	20	16	(80)	1	(5)	3	(15)
Total	**352**	**229**	**(65)**	**92**	**(26)**	**31**	**(9)**

The occurrence of LM in NHL may be seen at the time of initial diagnosis, at relapse, or at any time during the course of the systemic disease. In a review by Recht *et al.* of 156 patients with NHL at Memorial Sloan-Kettering Cancer Center, CNS disease was present at initial diagnosis in 27%, at relapse in 26%, and during the course of progressive systemic disease in 47%.[8] In a more recent retrospective review by Bollen *et al.* of

532 patients with NHL, only 11 patients presented with CNS disease and 55 patients developed CNS disease at relapse.[9] Bishop *et al.* found six among 23 patients with primary mediastinal thymic large B-cell lymphoma (PMLCL) who developed CNS disease.[7] The investigators selected this subset of patients from those with NHL because it has a high propensity for extranodal involvement of disease, a factor which has been reported as a reliable predictor of CNS disease. Two of the 23 patients (9%) presented with CNS disease at diagnosis; four patients (27%) developed CNS disease at relapse. Only one of the six patients had parenchymal disease without suggestion of LM.

2.2 Risk factors

Since the overall incidence of CNS disease is not sufficiently high enough to warrant CNS prophylaxis in all patients with NHL, it is important to identify those patients at an increased risk. Patients with identifiable risk factors for CNS disease may benefit from CNS prophylactic treatment. Various factors have been identified for the risk of CNS disease in NHL. These risk factors include: 1) lymphoma grade and stage, 2) extent of extranodal disease, 3) young age and, 4) elevated serum lactate dehydrogenase (LDH) levels. The relative importance of any of these individual risk factors has not been clearly identified in the literature.

Most series reveal an increased incidence of LM in NHL in patients with a high-grade lymphoma (Stage 4B) and a diffuse, lymphoblastic histology. In a review of 602 patients where there was an overall incidence of LM of 6.3%, Ersboll found that the highest frequency of LM was in the lymphoblastic histologic subtype (23%), compared to follicular small cleaved and mixed cell (1.6%), diffuse small cleaved cell (2.4%), and large cell immunoblastic (4.5%).[10] Litman also found an increased risk of CNS disease in patients with a diffuse histology (16 %) compared to those with nodular types (3%) in a series of 292 patients with NHL and an overall rate of CNS disease of 11%.[11]

The risk of CNS disease is also clearly related to the lymphoma grade, with the higher grade lymphomas carrying an increased risk of disease. Bollen *et al.* reported the association between CNS disease and lymphoma grade as follows: high-grade (39%), intermediate grade (22%), and low-grade (7%).[9] In a multivariate analysis, high and intermediate grade NHL and advanced stage were independent risk factors for CNS disease. There were no cases of low-grade lymphoma in the 51 of 833 patients with CNS disease in the review by Liang et al.[12] In the Memorial Sloan-Kettering analysis, 67% of the cases with CNS involvement of lymphoma were stage IV at the time of diagnosis.[8]

Several investigators have found an increased risk of CNS disease in NHL in patients with extranodal involvement of the lymphoma in sites such as sinus or orbit, bone marrow, blood, gastrointestinal tract, and testes. Liang found an increased incidence of CNS involvement in patients with lymphoma involving the orbit (43%), testes (40%), peripheral blood (33%), bone (29%), nasal/paranasal sinuses (23%), and bone marrow (20%).[13,12] In a recent prospective analysis, van Besien *et al.* confirmed the importance of the previously stated risk factors in predicting rates of CNS recurrence; however, in a multivariate analysis, these investigators found that only involvement of more than one extranodal site and an increased LDH were independent predictors of CNS recurrence.[14] The Kaplan-Meier estimate of CNS recurrence at one year in 93 out of 605 patients with these two risk factors was 17.4% compared to 2.8% in the remaining 512 patients. The authors concluded that this data suggests that the risk of CNS recurrence is determined by disease extent and proliferation rather than by any particular disease location. Unlike previous retrospective studies, this review was a prospective analysis and included only those patients with large-cell and immunoblastic lymphoma whose CNS disease was the initial site of recurrence rather than presenting after systemic relapse. The authors noted the significance of this fact to be that in the latter group, CNS recurrence is an expression of end-stage disease and is not, therefore, predicted by the same risk factors.

2.3 Clinical presentation and diagnosis

The clinical presentation of LM in patients with NHL is similar to that seen in patients with LM from solid tumors. However, patients with hematologic malignancies present with a higher frequency of cranial nerve signs as initial manifestations of LM.[3] Since LM involve the entire neuroaxis, their clinical symptoms and signs are typically divided into three general groups: 1) cerebral hemispheres, 2) cranial nerves and, 3) spinal cord and nerve roots. The most frequent presenting symptoms/signs are mental status change and headache followed by cranial nerve palsy and focal weakness or numbness.

The diagnosis of LM in NHL includes the clinical evaluation for the above-mentioned features as well as the radiographic appearance on neuroimaging studies and examination of CSF from lumbar puncture. The appearance of LM on gadolinium-enhanced magnetic resonance imaging (MRI) in the patient with lymphoma is similar to that in the patient with LM from a solid malignancy (Fig.1). Cranial imaging may show sulcal, ependymal, or cisternal enhancement in addition to subarachnoid nodules and communicating hydrocephalus. Tumor may also be seen infiltrating cranial nerves, either as enhancement or enlargement of the nerve. A spine

MRI may show intradural enhancing nodules as well as linear enhancement, enlargement, or asymmetry of nerve roots. Abnormal neuroimaging findings are found in approximately 40-50% of patients with LM from hematologic malignancies, slightly lower than in solid tumor patients.[15,16,17]

All patients suspected of LM should undergo lumbar puncture. In addition to the routine analysis of CSF for chemistry (total protein and glucose levels) and cytology, the CSF of patients suspected of lymphomatous meningitis may be analyzed for the presence of tumor markers including B_2 microglobulin and LDH isoenzymes, clonality of cells utilizing flow cytometry, and the presence of tumor-derived DNA by polymerase chain reaction (PCR) technique.[18] Initial CSF cytology is frequently more sensitive in patients with LM from solid tumors than in those with LM from hematologic malignancies. However, repeat lumbar punctures more frequently increase the diagnostic accuracy of cytologic examination in patients with hematologic malignancies; three lumbar punctures are usually sufficient to establish a diagnosis of LM in 90% of patients.

When lymphocytes present in the CSF cannot be identified as malignant, the demonstration of monoclonality, or B-cell origin using immunotyping of lymphocytes, may confirm the diagnosis of malignant tumor in the CSF. Most NHLs are of B-cell origin; reactive lymphocytes are more frequently T-cell. However, NHL often induces a secondary reactive T-cell infiltration. An elevated level of beta-2 microglobulin in the CSF compared to the serum level has been shown to be associated with LM at initial diagnosis in patients with lymphoma or leukemia.[19] PCR examination of the CSF for tumor-derived DNA from the lymphoma cell of either B-cell or T-cell origin has a greater sensitivity for tumor detection compared to routine cytology.

2.4 Treatment and survival

Currently, the goal of treatment of LM is palliative which often improves or delays progression of neurologic symptoms and signs. The reported median survival after CNS recurrence in NHL ranges between two and six months. The treatment of LM from NHL includes craniospinal irradiation, traditional systemic chemotherapy, intrathecal chemotherapy, and high-dose chemotherapy with hematopoietic stem cell rescue. The reported median patient survival after the development of LM, from both solid and hematologic cancers, is six months.[20] Since most CNS disease in NHL occurs in the setting of advanced or relapsed systemic disease, control of local or systemic lymphoma is critical.

Several investigators have suggested that those patients with NHL identified as high risk for CNS disease should receive intrathecal prophylaxis with either methotrexate or cytosine arabinoside. However, there has not been a prospective review to demonstrate that patients at such risk might have a prolonged median survival with prophylactic treatment. Moreover, these retrospective studies have shown that patients who did receive either radiation therapy or intrathecal chemotherapy had only improvement or stabilization of their neurologic symptoms. In a Dutch study, Paulus reported that more than 80% of patients with LM from NHL showed clinical improvement in their symptoms after treatment with either intrathecal chemotherapy or radiation therapy; however, the median survival was 3 1/2 months, with a six-month survival of 32%.[21] Van Besien *et al.* reported that only one of six patients with intermediate grade lymphoma responded to intrathecal treatment, and the median survival of patients treated with intrathecal therapy was only 42 days.[14] In this review, radiation therapy resulted in immediate although transient responses in six of nine patients. In a review of 31 patients with LM from lymphoma, Yoshida *et al.* found that prophylactic treatment was successful only in those patients with systemically well-controlled disease and, therefore, control of systemic lymphoma is of great importance.[22]

Radiotherapy treatment of LM should be directed to regions of bulky or symptomatic disease as seen on neuroimaging studies.[23] Although radiotherapy may stabilize or delay progression of neurologic symptoms, it does not prolong survival. Macgrath *et al.* retrospectively examined the outcome of 41 patients with NHL and CNS disease all of whom received systemic therapy and intrathecal chemotherapy.[23] He found that there was no difference in the rate of CNS relapse or survival in those patients who received radiation from those who did not receive radiation. However, an increase in neurologic toxicity was noted in those patients who received radiation.

Treatment of LM in NHL with radiation therapy, standard chemotherapy, and intrathecal therapy is palliative. High-dose chemotherapy with autologous bone marrow transplantation is superior to standard-dose therapy and can be curative in patients with recurrent NHL. In a prospective study of 215 patients with systemic relapses of NHL, Philip *et al.* reported a five-year event-free survival rate for patients who received chemotherapy and transplantation as 46% compared to 12% for those patients who received chemotherapy without transplantation.[24] The role of high-dose chemotherapy and bone marrow transplantation for patients with NHL and secondary CNS disease is not known. The European Bone Marrow Transplant Lymphoma Registry data suggest the possibility for this treatment approach in patients with NHL and CNS disease.[25] This retrospective review of 62 patients with NHL and CNS relapse demonstrated that the five-year progression-free survival (PFS) was 42% in the 45 patients who underwent high-dose chemotherapy and bone marrow transplant after clearing of their CNS disease by standard pre-transplant regimens. The PFS was only 9% in the remaining 17 patients with residual CNS disease at the time of bone marrow transplant. Moreover, patients who received radiotherapy and intrathecal chemotherapy had better outcomes than those who did not. In a more recent review by Alvarnas et al, similar results were found.[13] They reported on 15 patients with NHL and CNS disease (two with primary CNS lymphoma, 13 with metastatic CNS disease). Prior to bone marrow transplant, all patients received intrathecal chemotherapy, 13 received CNS radiotherapy, and 14 received systemic chemotherapy. The actuarial five-year event-free survival was 46%, and overall survival was 41%. These studies suggest that high-dose chemotherapy and bone marrow transplantation can extend survival times in patients with CNS involvement from NHL if patients are cleared of their CNS disease prior to transplantation.

3. LYMPHOMA IN THE ACQUIRED IMMUNE DEFICIENCY SYNDROME PATIENT

The incidence of NHL in the Acquired Immune Deficiency Syndrome (AIDS) population has been increasing.[26] AIDS-related NHL is commonly associated with a high-grade histology as well as a high incidence of extranodal involvement. In particular, both meningeal disease and parenchymal CNS disease have been reported as common sites of extranodal disease. The incidence of LM in AIDS-related NHL has been reported as 35% and is frequently associated with predominantly high-grade lymphomas such as immunoblastic and small noncleaved lymphomas.[27]

The clinical presentation of LM in AIDS patients is similar to that in immunocompetent patients. The diagnosis of CNS disease also includes neuroimaging studies and CSF analysis. However, unlike immunocompetent patients, there is a strong association between AIDS-related NHL and the presence of Epstein-Barr virus (EBV) DNA in the CSF from these patients. Epstein-Barr virus DNA is present in the CSF in approximately 70-80% of AIDS-related NHL and in virtually 100% of cases of AIDS-related primary CNS lymphoma (PCNSL).[28,29,30] Therefore, all AIDS patients with NHL suspected of CNS disease should have their CSF analyzed for the presence of EBV DNA using PCR. The presence of EBV-DNA in the CSF is a strong predictor of LM in AIDS-related NHL. Some investigators have suggested that as the result of this association, those AIDS patients with NHL and positive PCR's for EBV in their CSF should receive prophylactic intrathecal chemotherapy for LM.[27]

The treatment and response rates for LM in AIDS-related NHL are similar to that in immunocompetent patients. Standard treatment regimens include systemic chemotherapy with the addition of craniospinal radiation and intrathecal chemotherapy. Most reviews have shown that this treatment is only palliative with survival times not dissimilar from LM in immunocompetent patients with NHL. In a recent review, Desai *et al.* propose that some patients with AIDS-related NHL and LM are potentially curable[30]. They report on seven patients with AIDS-related NHL and LM who received standard systemic chemotherapy, whole brain radiotherapy, and intrathecal therapy. Four of these seven patients survived more than one year.

PCNSL is a common malignancy in AIDS patients, with an incidence of 10% in this patient population. It is the most common brain tumor seen in AIDS patients.[27] Although the incidence of PCNSL has risen three-fold in the past two to three decades, there has been a strong decline in the incidence of AIDS-related PCNSL since the introduction of highly active antiretroviral therapy (HAART). This can be attributed to control of the viral infection and relative reconstitution of the immune system with HAART. As in immunocompetent patients, AIDS-related PCNSL frequently invades the leptomeninges. Previously, palliative whole-brain radiotherapy was the only treatment offered to these patients.[31] However, patients with a good performance status may be able to tolerate combined modality therapy and have an improved outcome.[32,33]

4. LEUKEMIA

4.1 Pediatric acute lymphoblastic leukemia

With modern therapy, the event-free survival of pediatric patients with ALL is approximately 80%.[34] Prior to the inclusion of prophylactic therapy for CNS disease in the treatment of children with ALL, the major obstacle to cure was relapse of disease in the CNS. Meningeal relapse is a poor prognostic indicator of survival because it is typically followed by bone marrow relapse.[35] With new advances in the treatment of children with ALL, including CNS prophylaxis, the incidence of CNS relapse is now 5-10%.[36] An increased awareness of the neurologic toxicities of CNS irradiation in the pediatric patient has also led to a growing emphasis on prophylactic chemotherapy-based treatment regimens.

Various risk factors for the development of CNS disease in pediatric ALL have been identified. These risk factors include: 1) No CNS prophylaxis at the time of disease presentation, 2) an elevated white blood cell count, 3) the presence of blast cells in the cytospin preparation of the CSF, 4) an elevated serum LDH, 5) an elevated serum alkaline phosphatase, 6) a high proliferative index, 7) extramedullary disease, 8) age less than one year and, 9) the ALL sub-groups T-cell ALL and pro-B ALL. These risk factors have been used by clinicians to stratify children with ALL into low, intermediate, and high-risk groups for the development of CNS disease. Smith *et al.*, and the Cancer Therapy Evaluation Program of the National Cancer Institute, reviewed outcome data from pediatric patients in ALL clinical trials in order to define a uniform approach to risk classification.[37] They identified a standard-risk category composed of those patients with B-precursor ALL (age one to nine years), and white blood count less than 50,000/microL at diagnosis. The remaining patients were classified as high-risk ALL. The four-year event-free survival rate for the standard risk group was 80% versus 65% for the high-risk group.

The diagnosis of LM in patients with ALL is based upon CSF analysis and neuroimaging studies. The diagnosis requires the appearance of lymphoblasts in the CSF. Most investigators have established a standard of diagnosis which uses both the cell count and the presence of blast cells in the CSF. A cell count greater than five mononuclear cells per mm^3 CSF, as well as the identification of lymphoblasts in the cytospin preparation, are regarded as absolute criteria for the diagnosis of CNS disease.[38] In some cases, the CSF diagnosis may be difficult to establish. In others, the CSF may contain a high number of blast cells, but have a cell count less than 5 mm^3. In a multivariate analysis, Mahmoud *et al.* found that the presence of blast cells in the CSF in patients with less than five leukocytes per microliter was an independent risk factor of CNS relapse. In addition, these patients had a five-year probability of survival-free relapses confined to the CNS, lower than in patients whose CSF did not contain blast cells.[39] Another diagnostic difficulty may occur when the CSF sample contains blood. In this situation, the ratio of serum to CSF lymphoblasts should be considered.

Children with ALL most often have clinically silent leptomeningeal disease diagnosed by lumbar puncture. When symptoms do occur, they are identical to other patients with leptomeningeal lymphoma and include headache, nausea, cranial nerve palsies, radicular pain and weakness. In a review of 83 children with ALL, Ritchey et al found that 75% of the patients were asymptomatic at the time of diagnosis of CNS disease.[36]

Approximately 10 % of children with ALL will develop leukostasis (white blood count greater than 100,000/microL). The leukostasis is due to an impedance of blood flow secondary to intravascular clumping of white blood cells. Children with leukostasis have an increased risk of CNS disease and will often present with mental status changes and cranial nerve palsies.

Since CNS relapse in children with ALL predisposes the patient to bone marrow relapse and a poor clinical outcome, treatment of LM in these patients is primarily prophylactic. Studies of children with ALL and CNS relapse treated in the 1970's and 1980's report remission rates of 25-50%,[35,40] in comparison to those in more recent years of 70-80%.[36] This improvement in clinical outcome is largely due to the utilization of more intensive chemotherapy regimens. These treatment regimens include high-dose systemic chemotherapy with agents that penetrate the blood-brain barrier as well as intrathecal chemotherapy. CNS radiotherapy is often deferred to both minimize bone marrow toxicity, which may interfere with successful chemotherapy administration, and diminish neurotoxicity. The treatment approach is different for patients identified as low or intermediate risk compared to those identified as high-risk patients (see below). However, regardless of the patient's risk identification, treatment should be initiated at the time of diagnosis since most CNS relapse occurs within two years from the time of diagnosis.

Some of the earliest clinical trials were performed by the Berlin-Frankfurt-Munster Study Group and involved over 3500 patients since 1981.[40] They demonstrated that intensive systemic chemotherapy, in combination with intrathecal chemotherapy without CNS radiation, can prevent CNS disease in pediatric patients with ALL. In an initial trial, 279 children with ALL identified as low and intermediate risk were randomized to receive either cranial radiation (18 Gy) and intrathecal (IT) methotrexate or systemic methotrexate and IT methotrexate without radiotherapy. The investigators found a higher number of CNS relapses in the group of patients who did not receive cranial radiation in comparison to those who did (19 vs 3 patients). However, 16 of the 19 patients with CNS disease were in the intermediate risk group. Therefore, the replacement of cranial radiation with systemic methotrexate was only effective in the low-risk group of patients. Other investigators have reported similar results in treating low-risk patients with IT chemotherapy and standard systemic chemotherapy alone.[41,42]

In order to obtain similar treatment outcomes in the intermediate-risk patient, investigators have found that the avoidance of CNS radiotherapy requires an extended use of IT chemotherapy throughout induction, consolidation, and maintenance in combination with more intensive systemic chemotherapy. The Children's Cancer Group designed a prospective randomized trial to determine if IT methotrexate administered during induction, consolidation, and maintenance could provide prophylaxis from CNS disease equivalent to that of cranial radiation in children with ALL identified as intermediate-risk.[42] In this prospective randomized trial of 1,388 patients, the investigators found that the event-free survival rates for patients who received either cranial radiation or IT methotrexate in combination with systemic chemotherapy were 68 and 64%, respectively. Moreover, patients who received more intensive systemic chemotherapy had a 94% CNS relapse-free survival rate with either cranial radiotherapy or IT methotrexate, while patients who received standard systemic chemotherapy had 90% and 80% rates for radiotherapy and IT methotrexate, respectively.

Patients who are identified as high-risk for CNS relapse have a poor initial or delayed response to treatment, or have T-cell ALL requiring cranial radiation in addition to intensified systemic chemotherapy and IT chemotherapy.[43,44] Survival rates are improved in high-risk ALL children who have a slow response to initial systemic chemotherapy and who receive augmented post-induction chemotherapy rather than standard therapy.[45]

4.2 Adult acute lymphoblastic leukemia

Approximately 80% of patients with adult acute lymphoblastic leukemia (ALL) can achieve remissions with current treatment regimens. However, the cure rate remains low at 20-30%.[46,47] Extramedullary disease is common in adult patients with ALL and the CNS is a frequent location. At the time of diagnosis of ALL, LM are seen in 6% of adult patients with a range of 1-10%. The rate of relapse into the CNS is higher at approximately 30%.[46,47] As in pediatric patients with ALL, CNS relapse is frequently followed by bone marrow relapse and confers poor survival rates. The use of CNS prophylactic treatment can lower this incidence of CNS relapse and offer a better prognosis. It is generally recommended in all patients with ALL.

In an extensive review of the literature of the treatment of adult patients with ALL, Cortes found that approximately 60-70% of all adult patients with ALL have poor prognostic features[47]. These patients have a cure rate of 20-25% compared to 60-70% for those patients without such features. These poor prognostic features include advanced age, a high leukocyte count, a non-T-cell immunophenotype, Ph-positive genotype, and a longer time to achieve a complete remission. Patients with these risk factors may benefit from allogeneic bone marrow transplantation during first remission, in contrast to low risk patients who benefit from bone marrow transplant only at relapses.

In a retrospective literature review of 4000 adult patients with ALL, Gokbuget summarized the various prophylactic treatment approaches and their respective rates of CNS relapse.[48] These results demonstrated that the early administration of IT methotrexate in combination with CNS radiation, along with the continuation of IT treatment throughout maintenance therapy, is essential in order to provide the lowest rate of CNS relapse. In this review, the most significant risk factor for CNS relapse was the lack of CNS prophylaxis at the time of diagnosis. The neurologic toxicities of CNS radiation are not as severe in the adult ALL patient as in the pediatric ALL patient. The primary concern in the adult patient is bone marrow suppression and its consequences in combination with induction chemotherapy. There is a risk of leukoencephalopathy when radiation is used in combination with methotrexate. In trials with delayed radiation in adults, the risk of CNS relapse was 20% in comparison to 11% when radiation was used early.

Although bone marrow transplant is the most effective treatment in adult ALL patients who have sustained a CNS relapse, it is primarily directed towards the prevention of further bone marrow disease and, therefore, additional CNS treatment is also required. In a study of 198 patients with ALL treated with bone marrow transplant, the rate of CNS relapse was 52% in those patients without IT prophylaxis in contrast to 17% in patients who received IT methotrexate after transplant.[49]

5. CHRONIC LEUKEMIAS

Chronic lymphocytic leukemia (CLL) is the most common form of leukemia representing approximately 30% of all leukemias.[50] Chronic myelogenous leukemia (CML) accounts for 7-15% of leukemias in adults.[50] Both leukemias have an initial chronic phase which transforms into an accelerated and blastic phase. The prognosis of patients in the blastic phase is poor with low response rates to treatment and a median survival of only two to three months.[51] Leptomeningeal disease in both CLL and CML is extremely rare and, when it does occur, presents during the blastic phase of the disease. In a literature review of LM in CLL, Morrison found only 21 cases through 1998.[52] Patients have presenting symptoms similar to those of LM in the acute leukemias. These include headache, mental status change, and cranial nerve palsies. The diagnosis is made by the presence of leukemic cells in the CSF. Treatment regimens used are IT methotrexate and adjuvant CNS radiation, or CNS radiation alone. The majority of patients will have a treatment response if therapy is administered promptly at the time of diagnosis. However, survival rates are poor and prolonged remission is rare.

6. CONCLUSIONS

LM from hematologic malignancies are relatively similar to those from solid tumors in their clinical presentation, diagnosis, and poor prognostic indication of survival. Unlike solid tumors, LM from lymphoma and leukemia often are the initial presentation of cancer or occur during disease remission. At the present time, combined modality treatment of LM from hematologic malignancies with systemic and IT chemotherapy, cranial radiation, and bone marrow transplantation does not extend overall survival. However, when CNS prophylactic treatment is initiated early in patients identified as high risk for CNS disease, the rate of CNS relapse may be reduced and the development of neurologic symptoms delayed.

REFERENCES

1. DeAngelis LM. Current diagnosis and treatment of leptomeningeal metastasis. J Neurooncol 1998; 38:245-52.
2. Kaplan JG, DeSouza TG, Farkash A, et al. Leptomeningeal metastases: Comparison of clinical features and laboratory data of solid tumors, lymphomas and leukemias. J Neurooncol 1990; 9:225-9.
3. van Oostenbrugge RJ, Twijnstra A. Presenting features and value of diagnostic procedures in leptomeningeal metastases. Neurology 1999; 53:382-5.
4. Freedman A, Nadler LM. Non-Hodgkin's Lymphomas. In : Cancer Medicine, 4th Edition, 1997. Holland J, Bast RC JR, Morton ML, Frei E III, Kufe DW, Weichselbaum RR (Eds). Williams & Wilkins, Baltimore, pp 2757-2795.
5. Cuttner J, Meyer R, Huang YP. Intercranial involvement in Hodgkin's disease. A report of 6 cases and review of the literature. Cancer 1979; 43:1497-1506.
6. Perez-Jaffe LA, Salhany KE, Green RJ, et al. Cerebral spinal fluid involvement by Hodgkin's disease diagnosed by CSF cytology and immunocytochemistry. Diagn Cytopathol 1999; 20:219-223.
7. Bishop PC, Wilson WH, Pearson D, et al. CNS involvement in primary mediastinal large B-cell lymphoma. J Clin Oncol 1999; 17:2479-85.
8. Recht L, Straus DJ, Cirrincione C, Thaler HT, Posner JB. Central nervous system metastases from non-Hodgkin's lymphoma: Treatment and prophylaxis. Am J Med 1988; 84:425-35.
9. Bollen EL, Brouwer RE, Hamers S, et al. Central nervous system relapse in non-Hodgkin's lymphoma. A single-center study of 532 patients. Arch Neurol 1997; 54:854-9.
10. Ersboll J, Schultz HB, Thomsen BL, Keiding N, Nissen NI. Meningeal involvement in non-Hodgkin's lymphoma: symptoms, incidence, risk factors and treatment. Scand J Haematol 1985; 35:487-96.
11. Litam JP, Cabanillas F, Smith TL, Bodey GP, Freireich EJ. Central nervous system relapse in malignant lymphomas: risk factors and implications for prophylaxis. Blood 1979; 54:1249-57.
12. Liang R, Chiu E, Loke SL. Secondary central nervous system involvement by non-Hodgkin's lymphoma: the risk factors. Hematol Oncol 1990; 8:141-5.
13. Alvarnas JC, Negrin RS, Horning SJ, et al. High-dose therapy with hematopoietic cell transplantation for patients with central nervous system involvement by non-Hodgkin's lymphoma. Biol Blood Marrow Transplant 2000; 6:352-8.
14. van Besien K, Ha CS, Murphy S, et al. Risk factors, treatment, and outcome of central nervous system recurrence in adults with intermediate-grade and immunoblastic lymphoma. Blood 1998; 91:1178-84.

15. Gomori JM, Heching N, Siegal T. Leptomeningeal metastases: evaluation by gadolinium enhanced spinal magnetic resonance imaging. J Neurooncol 1998; 36:55-60.
16. Collie DA, Sellar RJ, Steyn JP, Cull RE. The diagnostic yield of magnetic resonance imaging (MRI) of the brain and spine requested by general practitioners: comparison with hospital clinicians. Br J Gen Pract 1999; 49:559-61.
17. Chamberlain M. Leptomeningeal Metastases. In: Cancer in the Nervous System. Levin V (Ed.), Churchill Livingstone, New York, 1996, pp 282-290.
18. Rhodes CH, Glantz MJ, Glantz L,et al. A comparison of polymerase chain reaction examination of cerebrospinal fluid and conventional cytology in the diagnosis of lymphomatous meningitis. Cancer 1996; 77:543-8.
19. Jeffery GM, Frampton CM, Legge HM, Hart DN. Cerebrospinal fluid B2-microglobulin levels in meningeal involvement by malignancy. Pathology 1990; 22:20-3.
20. Chamberlain MC. Leptomeningeal metastases: A review of evaluation and treatment. J Neurooncol 1998; 37:271-84.
21. Paulus JA, Bos GM, Lowenberg B, Van Den Bent MJ. Treatment results and the prognosis in patients with localization of non-Hodgkin's lymphoma in the central nervous system. Ned Tijdschr Geneeskd 1998; 142:2196-200.
22. Yoshida S, Morii K, Watanabe M, Saito T. Characteristic features of malignant lymphoma with central nervous system involvement. Surg Neurol 2000;53:163-7.
23. Magrath IT, Haddy TB, Adde MA. Treatment of patients with high-grade non-Hodgkin's lymphomas and central nervous system involvement: is radiation an essential component of therapy? Leuk Lymphoma 1996; 21:99-105.
24. Philip T, Guglielmi C, Hagenbeek A, et al. Autologous bone marrow transplantation as compared with salvage chemotherapy in relapses of chemotherapy-sensitive non-Hodgkin's lymphoma. N Engl J Med 1995; 333:1540-5.
25. Williams CD, Pearce R, Taghipour G, et al. Autologous bone marrow transplantation for patients with non-Hodgkin's lymphoma and CNS involvement: Those transplanted with active CNS disease have a poor outcome--a report by the European Bone Marrow Transplant Lymphoma Registry. J Clin Oncol 1994; 12:2415-22.
26. Rabkin CS, Yellin F. Cancer incidence in a population with a high prevalence of infection with human immunodeficiency virus type 1. J Natl Cancer Inst 1994; 86:1711-6.
27. Taiwo BO. AIDS-related primary CNS lymphoma: A brief review. AIDS Read 2000; 10:486-91.
28. Cingolani A, Gastaldi R, Fassone L, et al. Epstein-Barr virus infection is predictive of CNS involvement in systemic AIDS-related non-Hodgkin's lymphomas. J Clin Oncol 2000; 18:3325-30.
29. DeAngelis LM, Wong E, Rosenblum M, Furneaux H. Epstein-Barr virus in acquired immune deficiency syndrome (AIDS) and non-AIDS primary central nervous system lymphoma. Cancer 1992; 70:1607-11.
30. Desai J, Mitnick RJ, Henry DH, Llena J, Sparano JA. Patterns of central nervous system recurrence in patients with systemic human immunodeficiency virus-associated non-Hodgkin's lymphoma. Cancer 1999; 86:1840-7.
31. Goldstein JD, Dickson DW, Moser FG, et al. Primary central nervous system lymphoma in acquired immune deficiency syndrome. A clinical and pathologic study with results of treatment with radiation. Cancer 1991; 67:2756-65.
32. Raez LE, Patel P, Feun L, et al. Natural history and prognostic factors for survival in patients with acquired immune deficiency syndrome (AIDS)-related primary central nervous system lymphoma (PCNSL). Crit Rev Oncol 1998; 9:199-208.
33. Chamberlain MC, Kormanik PA. AIDS-related central nervous system lymphomas. J Neurooncol 1999; 43:269-76.

34. Mahoney DH Jr, Shuster JJ, Nitschke R, et al. Intensification with intermediate-dose intravenous methotrexate is effective therapy for children with lower-risk B-precursor acute lymphoblastic leukemia: A Pediatric Oncology Group study. J Clin Oncol 2000; 18:1285-94.

35. Ortega JA, Nesbit ME, Sather HN, et al. Long-term evaluation of a CNS prophylaxis trial--treatment comparisons and outcome after CNS relapse in childhood ALL: A report from the Childrens Cancer Study Group. J Clin Oncol 1987; 5:1646-54.

36. Ritchey AK, Pollock BH, Lauer SJ, et al. Improved survival of children with isolated CNS relapse of acute lymphoblastic leukemia: A pediatric oncology group study. J Clin Oncol 1999; 17:3745-52.

37. Smith M, Arthur D, Camitta B, et al. Uniform approach to risk classification and treatment assignment for children with acute lymphoblastic leukemia. J Clin Oncol 1996; 14:18-24.

38. Schrappe M, Reiter A, Riehm H. Prophylaxis and treatment of neoplastic meningeosis in childhood acute lymphoblastic leukemia. J Neurooncol 1998; 38:159-65.

39. Mahmoud HH, Rivera GK, Hancock ML, et al. Low leukocyte counts with blast cells in cerebrospinal fluid of children with newly diagnosed acute lymphoblastic leukemia. N Engl J Med 1993; 329:314-9.

40. Schrappe M, Beck J, Brandeis WE, et al. Treatment of acute lymphoblastic leukemia in childhood and adolescence: results of the multicenter therapy study ALL-BFM 81. Klin Padiatr 1987; 199:133-50.

41. Pullen J, Boyett J, Shuster J, et al. Extended triple intrathecal chemotherapy trial for prevention of CNS relapse in good-risk and poor-risk patients with B-progenitor acute lymphoblastic leukemia: a Pediatric Oncology Group study. J Clin Oncol 1993; 11:839-49.

42. Tubergen DG, Gilchrist GS, O'Brien RT, et al. Prevention of CNS disease in intermediate-risk acute lymphoblastic leukemia: Comparison of cranial radiation and intrathecal methotrexate and the importance of systemic therapy: A Childrens Cancer Group report. J Clin Oncol 1993; 11:520-6.

43. Conter V, Arico M, Valsecchi MG, et al. Long-term results of the Italian Association of Pediatric Hematology and Oncology (AIEOP) acute lymphoblastic leukemia studies, 1982-1995. Leukemia 2000; 14:2196-204.

44. Nachman J, Sather HN, Cherlow JM, et al. Response of children with high-risk acute lymphoblastic leukemia treated with and without cranial irradiation: A report from the Children's Cancer Group. J Clin Oncol 1998; 16:920-30.

45. Nachman JB, Sather HN, Sensel MG, et al. Augmented post-induction therapy for children with high-risk acute lymphoblastic leukemia and a slow response to initial therapy. N Engl J Med 1998; 338:1663-71.

46. Hoelzer DF. Therapy of the newly diagnosed adult with acute lymphoblastic leukemia. Hematol Oncol Clin North Am 1993; 7:139-60.

47. Cortes JE, Kantarjian HM. Acute lymphoblastic leukemia. A comprehensive review with emphasis on biology and therapy. Cancer 1995; 76:2393-417.

48. Gokbuget N, Hoelzer D. Meningeosis leukemia in adult acute lymphoblastic leukaemia. J Neurooncol 1998; 38:167-80.

49. Thompson CB, Sanders JE, Flournoy N, Buckner CD, Thomas ED. The risks of central nervous system relapse and leukoencephalopathy in patients receiving marrow transplants for acute leukemia. Blood 1986; 67:195-9.

50. Cortes J, Aguayo A, Kantarjian H. Chronic leukemias. In: Cancer Management: A Multidisciplinary Approach. Pazdur R, Coia LR, Hoskins WJ, Wagmen LD (Eds.) PRR, Melville, NY, 2000, pp 657-680.

51. Sacchi S, Kantarjian HM, O'Brien S, et al. Chronic myelogenous leukemia in nonlymphoid blastic phase: Analysis of the results of first salvage therapy with three different treatment approaches for 162 patients. Cancer 1999; 86:2632-41.
52. Morrison C, Shah S, Flinn IW. Leptomeningeal involvement in chronic lymphocytic leukemia. Cancer Pract 1998; 6:223-8.

Chapter 5

LEPTOMENINGEAL METASTASIS OF PRIMARY CENTRAL NERVOUS SYSTEM (CNS) NEOPLASMS

Herbert H. Engelhard, M.D., Ph.D. and Luke A. Corsten, M.D.
The University of Illinois at Chicago, Chicago, Illinois

Abstract: Leptomeningeal dissemination of primary CNS tumors varies widely by histologic subtype. In certain tumors including medulloblastoma, ependymoma, germ cell tumors, and primary CNS lymphoma, seeding of the cerebrospinal fluid space is a critical factor in determining stage, prognosis and appropriate therapy. Other tumor types, such as glioma, may have radiographic evidence of leptomeningeal metastases without clear impact on prognosis or therapy.

Key Words: Medulloblastoma; ependymoma; glioma; primary CNS lymphoma; leptomeningeal metastases

1. INTRODUCTION

As discussed in previous chapters, many types of malignant tumors originating outside the central nervous system (CNS) are known to metastasize to the leptomeninges, including lymphomas, leukemias, and carcinomas from various primary sites. The spread of primary CNS neoplasms through the leptomeningeal space may be a fairly frequent occurrence, but has not been thoroughly studied, especially in adults. In 1837, Ollivier reported the autopsy findings of a patient with a cerebellar tumor that had spread throughout the leptomeningeal space of the cisterna magna, referring to it as "sarcomatous meningitis".[1] This likely represents the first reported case of a primary CNS tumor with leptomeningeal metastasis (LM).

The propensity of medulloblastomas to spread via cerebrospinal fluid (CSF) pathways was known in the mid- to late 1800's, and was well described in the early 1900's by Cushing.[2] While the classification of primary CNS tumors is extensive,[3] a medulloblastoma is an embryonal tumor of the posterior fossa and in a category that is distinct from the gliomas, the major sub-categories of which include astrocytoma, oligodendroglioma and ependymoma.[2-5]

Dissemination of high-grade glioma cells through the leptomeningeal space can be termed "leptomeningeal gliomatosis".[6] Primary diffuse leptomeningeal gliomatosis (PDLG) is an extremely rare disease entity which shares features with LM from CNS neoplasms. Patients usually present with non-focal symptoms, such as headache or seizures, then experience a progressive, downhill clinical course.[7,8] Alterations of mental status, papilledema, hydrocephalus, meningismus, cranial nerve palsies and symptoms and signs from spinal involvement may also be seen. With this disease, no distinct primary tumor (or source for the seeding) can be found, even at autopsy. While magnetic resonance imaging (MRI) may show meningeal enhancement with gadolinium, CSF cytology is usually negative.

In patients with PDLG, biopsy of an enhancing area of the meninges may lead to diagnosis.[9] Treatment is usually not very effective, although a complete remission in one case has been reported with the use of cortico-spinal radiation, multidrug systemic chemotherapy, ventricular and lumbar shunting, and intrathecal methotrexate.[9] In PDLG, malignant cells are presumed to arise from ectopic rests of glial tissue outside the pial plane of the CNS with resultant dissemination along the leptomeninges.[7,8] Varying lineages of glial cells may be involved, and the disease may occur anywhere within the leptomeningeal space.[7] PDLG has even been reported to be a cause of "sudden death".[10] As imaging of the neuroaxis improves, smaller primary sites may be detected and the diagnosis of PDLG may become even more rare.

The meninges themselves (leptomeninges and pachymeninges) can give rise to both malignant and benign tumors (such as meningiomas).[3] The propensity for even benign meningiomas to spread along the dura (and thus the need to resect infiltrated dura along with tumor removal) is well known. Primary leptomeningeal lymphoma is a rare primary tumor of the leptomeninges.[11] In this chapter, several topics will be reviewed including: 1) the possible mechanisms of leptomeningeal spread from CNS tumors, 2) the spectrum of CNS tumors found to lead to LM, both in children and adults, 3) the incidence of LM from CNS tumors, 4) the clinical presentation and diagnostic evaluation of these patients and, 5) treatment options, follow-up measures and prognosis.

2. MECHANISMS OF METASTASIS

In the literature, three different pathways have been suggested through which cells from a CNS tumor might gain access to the leptomeningeal space.[12-15] First, a tumor might be in direct contact with the CSF pathways, as in the case of a medulloblastoma or intraventricular tumor. In this situation, tumor cells could be "shed" directly into the CSF. Second, tumor cells might invade the leptomeningeal space by moving through and or displacing normal brain parenchyma, then eroding through the pia mater or ependyma, i.e. direct extension. This is currently believed to be the most likely mechanism through which tumors gain access to the leptomeningeal space. Proximity to the CSF pathways would then be a "risk factor" for the occurrence of such erosion, and dissemination. Nishio et al performed an autopsy study of 26 patients with different types of brain tumors and found that focal ependymal defects were often present, especially in patients with hydrocephalus.[16] A third possibility is that tumor cells might be directly "inoculated" into the CSF at the time of a surgical procedure, such as a craniotomy or CSF shunt.

Many years ago, support for the "surgical inoculation" theory was found in studies which examined the proportion of preoperative versus postoperative CSF samples with positive cytology in patients undergoing surgery for medulloblastoma.[12] More recently, Elliott and colleagues did a retrospective review of 51 patients with malignant glioma studying both surgical entry into the ventricle, and proximity of the tumor to the ventricular system, on CSF tumor dissemination and survival. Neither dissemination nor survival were found to be influenced either by ventricular entry during surgery or proximity of the tumor to the ventricular system. Survival rate was significantly decreased, however, once CSF tumor dissemination had occurred.[17] LM can occur even in the absence of surgical intervention. In current neurosurgical practice, while it is recognized that entering various CSF compartments could potentially lead to seeding, it is not felt that such maneuvers have a clinically significant negative impact.

Little data is available which directly pertains to the molecular mechanisms through which CNS tumors might gain access to, and disseminate through, the leptomeningeal space. Most of the current understanding is based on extrapolation from *in vitro* and *in vivo* studies of cultured glioblastoma cells. Malignant glioma cells are believed to be highly mobile,[18,19,20] in addition to being able to proliferate rapidly. They can secrete a variety of proteases including urokinase (also called urokinase-type plasminogen activator, or u-PA), matrix metalloproteinases, and/or lysosomal cysteine peptidases called cathepsins.[21,22,23,24,25] Such proteases facilitate the processes of migration and invasion by causing breakdown of the extracellular matrix and other physiologic microstructures within the CNS. Evidence also suggests that altered expression of certain membrane adhesion molecules (such as CD44 or cadherins) correlates with a tumor's ability to invade pial, arachnoid, ependymal, or even endothelial barriers.[26,12,28,29] Such phenotypic characteristics are likely to be important prerequisites for the metastatic process.

3. CNS TUMOR TYPES LEADING TO LM: CHILDREN AND ADULTS

The high tendency for several types of childhood brain tumors to metastasize to the leptomeninges has long been recognized. In addition to medulloblastoma, these tumors include ependymoma, germinoma, pineoblastoma and other primitive neuroectodermal tumors (PNETs).[2,4,15,30,31,32,33] The leptomeningeal spread of pediatric posterior fossa tumors has been especially well-documented.[15,30,32,34,35,37] The known propensity of these tumors to lead to "drop metastases", i.e. metastases to the spinal subarachnoid space, has resulted in standard protocols for CSF analysis, staging of the entire neuraxis with gadolinium enhanced MRI, and the administration of cranio-spinal irradiation. Leptomeningeal spread has been reported to occur with other pediatric brain tumors, including juvenile pilocytic astrocytomas, brainstem and other gliomas, and tumors of the choroid plexus.[14,15,32,26,38-48] CNS tumors that have been found to produce LM both in children and adults are listed in Table 1. It should be noted that in Table 1, no particular order has been assigned and many of the tumor types listed are from single case reports, or very small series.

Table 1. Primary CNS Tumors Reported to Produce Leptomeningeal Metastases

Children	**Adults**
Medulloblastoma	Glioblastoma
Ependymoma (benign and malignant)	Grade III astrocytoma
Germ cell tumors	Germ cell tumors
Pineoblastoma	Ependymoma
Primitive neuroectodermal tumor (PNET)	PNET
Juvenile pilocytic astrocytoma	Oligodendroglioma
Brainstem glioma	Low-grade glioma
Pleomorphic xanthoastrocytoma	Craniopharyngioma
High-grade glioma (other)	Malignant (and clear cell) meningioma
Choroid plexus papilloma/carcinoma	Primary cerebral fibrosarcoma
Ganglioglioma	Pituitary adenoma
Polar spongioblastoma	Pineoblastoma
Spinal cord astrocytoma	PNET
	Central neurocytoma
	Dermoid/epidermoid
	Primary CNS lymphoma
	Meningeal hemangiopericytoma
	Primary diffuse leptomeningeal gliomatosis

For adults, review of the literature reveals reports of LM from both low and high grade primary CNS tumors of varying cell lineages.[5,46,49,50-68] While the adult list is similar to that for children, the predominant histologies responsible for LM in adults are generally of higher grade, a reflection of the more frequent occurrence of these types of tumors in adults. More benign tumors more often have a longer interval between their initial diagnosis and the diagnosis of LM. Recurrent tumors and malignant tumors are generally more likely to be associated with LM. Spinal cord tumors have also been reported to lead to LM, including intracranial seeding, both in children and adults.[13,69-72]

4. INCIDENCE OF LM FROM CNS TUMORS

In series of children with brain tumors, the incidence of LM has ranged from 19% to 36%.[15,30,32,] With respect to specific tumor types, in 1983 Tomita and McLone reported that five out of five patients with cerebellar medulloblastoma had neoplastic cells present in the CSF or arachnoid of the cisterna magna at the time of craniotomy before manipulation of the tumor.[37] A more detailed study was then undertaken in which 31 children with medulloblastoma were studied by myelography and CSF cytology, one month after surgery, and prior to the administration of irradiation. Three patients (9.6%) showed results that were positive for spinal subarachnoid seeding.[34] The incidence of leptomeningeal metastasis in patients with medulloblastoma is known to vary with the age of the patient, with younger patients having a higher incidence of LM at time of diagnosis. The likelihood of LM is also known to vary with stage of the disease, e.g. initial diagnosis vs. tumor recurrence. In studying children with low-grade gliomas, Civitello et al found LM in one of 56 cerebellar tumors, one of 34 cerebral tumors, one of 21 chiasmatic tumors, 0 of 14 diencephalic tumors, and three of 12 spinal cord tumors.[40] The incidence of LM in children with brainstem gliomas has been reported to range from 4 to 33%.[46,62] Ependymomas, germ cell tumors and choroid plexus carcinomas are also known to frequently produce spinal seeding and/or "drop" metastases.[4,15,30,32,72]

For adults, Awad et al. reported a LM incidence of 7% in a series of 191 patients with supratentorial malignant gliomas.[50] Erlich and Davis found that 25% of 25 patients with glioblastoma had spinal LM as discerned at autopsy.[73] In another autopsy study of glioblastoma patients, Onda and colleagues found that 14 of 51 patients (27%) had dissemination of tumor cells into the CSF.[74] Clinical symptoms were found to be related to how extensive the seeding was. Wai-Kwan et al reported an incidence of 23% of LM in patients with malignant glioma as proven by autopsy.[67] In a study by

Elliott *et al.*, CSF dissemination could be radiographically documented in 35% of patients with malignant gliomas.[17] Schild et al reported leptomeningeal seeding in 10% of patients with benign ependymoma, and 41% in patients with malignant ependymoma.[33] In addition to tumor type and grade, the incidence of LM in adults may depend upon additional factors such as age and the extent of tumor spread at time of diagnosis.

In a recent study of 9672 patients of all ages having primary tumors of the brain or spinal cord, 11.5% had involvement of the cranial meninges and 2.2% had involvement of the CSF or spinal meninges. This study was based on patients collected through tumor registries; the diagnosis of meningeal and/or CSF involvement was made by clinical symptomatology and/or diagnostic imaging.[75] In contrast to studies cited above, Nishio and colleagues reported finding evidence for leptomeningeal seeding of the ventricular surface and/or subarachnoid space in 76.9% of the patients they studied.[16] Patients had a variety of primary CNS tumors, and were studied in detail at the time of autopsy. Malignant tumors showed tumor seeding more often than benign ones. In all of the cases in which seeding occurred, the primary tumor was found to extend directly into the CSF. The distribution of the tumor metastases correlated with CSF flow and the site of focal ependymal defects. Nishio et al. attributed their higher incidence to the fact that their patients were scrutinized more closely by detailed autopsy.

The fact that there is such a wide range of reported incidence rates, both in children and adults, is a product of the fact that the patients studied, and methods used, have varied from study to study. Analysis of patients for the occurrence of LM on clinical grounds is also clouded by the sometimes rapid progression of the primary tumor, with patients succumbing to the disease before the diagnosis of dissemination can be made. Therefore, uncertainty currently exists, as to the true incidence of LM.

5. DIAGNOSIS OF LM IN BRAIN TUMOR PATIENTS

The diagnosis of LM in general can be difficult to make, since patients may initially have vague complaints and minimal neurologic findings. LM may go on to mimic other disorders, such as tuberculosis or fungal meningitis, CNS sarcoidosis or pseudotumor cerebri.[10,31,76] As mentioned in the introduction of this chapter, lymphomatous meningitis and PDLG, primary neoplastic diseases of the leptomeninges, would present a similar picture. The diagnosis of LM for brain tumor patients can also be hampered by the vagueness of the symptoms that may be present, especially since the CNS is already involved with tumor. Occasionally, patients with primary brain tumors exhibit features of LM at the time of their initial presentation.[31,77] Multiple cranial nerve lesions as the initial manifestation of glioblastoma, for instance, is only rarely seen.[77]

Usually, for patients known to have a malignant brain tumor, there is little relevance to making the additional diagnosis of LM. This situation may change as treatment of the primary site improves. In patients for whom the diagnosis of LM has been important, such as pediatric medulloblastoma and ependymoma patients, more clinical research efforts have been focused.

Symptoms and signs of LM may be secondary to CSF obstruction and hydrocephalus (headache), cranial nerve involvement, involvement of the region of the fourth ventricle (intractable vomiting), irritation/compression of spinal nerve roots or spinal cord, or irritation of the cerebral cortex (seizures).[5,38,39,46,52,53,56,70,77] The key to the diagnosis of LM in a CNS tumor patient often lies in detecting symptoms and signs related to nervous system involvement in a new location. A typical scenario would be a patient with a supratentorial tumor presenting with new lower cranial nerve findings, or a cervical or lumbar radiculopathy. The extent of meningeal spread may be quite advanced by the time the diagnosis of LM is made. Table 2 shows a list of symptoms and signs that are possible in patients with LM; however, these findings may also be seen in patients with primary CNS tumors without LM.

Table 2. Possible Symptoms and Signs of Patients with Leptomeningeal Metastases

Cranial	Headache	Nausea
	Seizure	Nuchal rigidity
	Mental status changes	Papilledema
	Diplopia	Dysphagia
	Other cranial nerve palsies	
	Weakness	
	Intractable vomiting	
	Hypothalamic dysfunction	
Spinal	Back pain	Radiculopathy
	Myelopathy	Paralysis
	Incontinence	

Diagnostic studies such as MRI or computerized tomography (CT), with and without contrast media, are usually indicated at intervals for any patient with a known primary CNS tumor. Findings indicative or suspicious for LM include enhancement along the pial and/or ependymal (periventricular) surface (especially in a nodular pattern), obliteration of sulci or other structures normally containing CSF (such as the basal cisterns), and/or the occurrence of hydrocephalus. While T1 imaging is standard, T2 imaging may also be helpful. It is anticipated that in the future, with the availability of clinical MRI units having even higher field strengths, even smaller metastatic deposits will be detected. Additional techniques, such as diffusion tensor imaging are also becoming available and may prove to be of value.

The need for detailed imaging of the entire neuraxis, usually by MRI with and without gadolinium administration, depends on the patient's age, tumor type, clinical presentation and relevance of any positive findings. Proximity of the primary tumor to the ventricular system, other CSF pathways, or the pial surface of the brain or spinal cord would arouse suspicion for potential leptomeningeal seeding. Screening MRI scans of the entire spine are routinely performed for children with medulloblastoma, supratentorial PNET, ependymoma and germinoma. No such standards exist for adult patients with malignant gliomas. The reason for this seems to be the relatively low incidence of metastases and uncertain clinical significance of detecting LM in this population.

As mentioned above, leptomeningeal dissemination may cause hydrocephalus, and treatment (usually with a ventriculoperitoneal [VP] shunt) may be needed. It has been hypothesized that communicating and/or noncommunicating hydrocephalus could be caused in LM patients by: 1) mechanical obstruction of CSF pathways, 2) blockage of the sites of resorption of spinal fluid by tumor cells, either over the cerebral convexities or in the spinal subarachnoid space, 3) alteration of CSF viscosity due to increased protein content, and/or 4) increased fibrinogen in the CSF with conversion into fibrin (and fibrosis) at the basal cisterns and/or Pachionian granulations.[70] VP shunt placement may risk further spread of tumor cells, but this may be unavoidable since increased intracranial pressure from hydrocephalus may be fatal.

As with the clinical presentation of LM in general, CSF findings in patients with LM may be negative, or mimic those of other diseases. Standard CSF values in patients with LM from primary CNS tumors may be normal, or may show elevated protein, decreased glucose, increased cell number and/or positive malignant cells.[76] If the cell count is elevated, an increase in polymorphonuclear leukocytes may be seen. CSF cultures for fungus, and all other organisms would be expected to be negative. Performing a lumbar puncture in a patient with an intracranial mass lesion can certainly be hazardous; ventricular CSF may be available if the patient is requiring a VP shunt for hydrocephalus.

CSF cytology may be negative in patients with LM from CNS tumors, especially early in the clinical course.[31] In adults, studies attempting to correlate preoperative or postoperative CSF analysis with tumor diagnosis or degree of malignancy have not shown any reliable means for identifying those at risk for LM,[12,81] Balhuizen et al found positive preoperative CSF cytology in 13.9% of their glioma patients, although there was no correlation for risk of postoperative LM.[12] Sampling of CSF by lumbar puncture to document the presence or absence of malignant cells at the onset of treatment has been found to be of value in children. Positive CSF cytology has been shown to correlate with increased risk of gross LM and poorer overall prognosis. Negative CSF cytology, however, does not assure the absence of subsequent LM either in children or adults.[15,30]

6. TREATMENT AND PROGNOSIS FOR LM IN BRAIN TUMOR PATIENTS

Once the presence of LM from a brain tumor has been identified, options may include radiation therapy, systemic chemotherapy, and/or intra-thecal chemotherapy. Another option, especially for patients with leptomeningeal gliomatosis, is supportive care.[6] Choice of treatment depends on which treatments have already been administered, and the age and clinical status of the patient. Steroids, usually dexamethasone, may be given, or the dose increased to ameliorate symptoms. Patients who develop hydrocephalus may need a ventricular shunt.

Surgical intervention may be indicated at the site of tumor spread if a mass is present and prognosis is reasonable. Cases of drop metastases from CNS tumors (such as juvenile pilocytic astrocytomas and malignant meningiomas) have been treated with local surgical resection, especially when an isolated intra-dural metastasis has been present.[14,36,39,48,58,79] Surgical resection has also been combined with spinal irradiation. Stereotactic radiosurgery has long been used to provide a precise high-intensity boost of radiation in selected patients with recurrent intracranial tumors. With the development of new devices having the capability of performing radiosurgery of the spine (such as the CyberKnife™), this technology might also be attempted for selected patients with drop metastases.

Since the occurrence of LM in children with medulloblastomas, supratentorial PNETs, posterior fossa ependymomas, brainstem gliomas and germ cell tumors has been fairly well-defined, protocols for treatment with cranio-spinal radiation and/or chemotherapy have been developed.[4,12,15,32,35,43,46,80] The toxicities that are encountered may be quite significant. Often in the very young, every effort is made to attempt to avoid radiation therapy. Cranio-spinal radiation and/or chemotherapy have also been used to treat LM for more benign childhood tumors.[4,36,39,40,44,45,47,79] Controversies still exist concerning the indications for, and timing of, chemotherapy and radiation therapy in the pediatric age group. Follow-up measures for children with LM may include serial CSF analyses for cytology, and serial imaging studies, usually MRI with and without gadolinium administration.

In adults with malignant CNS tumors, the occurrence of LM despite chemotherapy and/or radiation has usually been addressed with additional radiation treatments and/or chemotherapy.[46,49,59,67] For LM from malignant glioma (intracranial or spinal), intrathecal chemotherapy with methotrexate, cytosine arabinoside (ara-C), thiotriethylenephosphoramide (thio-TEPA), neocarzinostatin or ACNU has also been tried.[6,53,62,69,82] Of these choices, thio-TEPA may be the most promising.[82] The potential toxic effect of intrathecal methotrexate administration is well known.[83] Adults are followed clinically for LM with serial neurologic examinations and MR imaging. For ventricular size, CT scanning is usually faster and less expensive than MRI. Follow-up CSF analysis is less likely to be of benefit in the adult population, and as mentioned above, lumbar puncture entails a risk of transtentorial herniation in the presence of supratentorial mass effect.

The prognosis for children with LM is variable, and depends upon the patient's tumor type, age, and extent of the tumor's spread at the time of diagnosis. Disease may progress despite neuraxis radiotherapy and intensive chemotherapy, and systemic metastases may occur.[31] In looking at pediatric patients with either medulloblastoma or PNET, Allen et al found the median survival for patients with LM at the time of diagnosis to be 12 months.[30] In a series review of 319 patients, Packer et al, found the median survival for patients, including all tumor types, to be six months.[15] Once there was evidence of relapse following treatment for LM, the median survival dropped to four months. When considering patients with the diagnosis of PNET, those with LM at the time of diagnosis fared worse than those without LM at the time of diagnosis, with an approximate five-year survival of 21% versus 54%.[15]. Civitello et al found the median survival for children diagnosed with low-grade gliomas and LM (combining all locations) to be only 25 months.[40] In looking at 14 patients with brainstem glioma and LM, Mantravadi et al found the five-year survival to be 28%.[62]

Unfortunately, the vast majority of adult patients with LM from primary CNS neoplasms have more aggressive tumor types and the prognosis is usually quite poor. Like children, prognosis may depend upon the type of the primary tumor, the age of the patient, and the extent of the tumor's spread. Wai-Kwan et al found that for patients with high-grade gliomas, the median survival for those with LM at the time of diagnosis was 49 weeks.[67] Awad et al reviewed 12 patients with high-grade glioma and LM at the time of diagnosis and found the average length of survival to be three months.[50]

Better treatments for LM, including LM from CNS tumors, are certainly needed.[6,84] The possibility of using immunotherapy for treating patients with

LM has always been attractive.[84] Coakham and Kemshead have reported on their experience with intrathecal administration of radiolabeled monoclonal antibodies.[85] Of note is the fact that the best results were obtained in patients with PNET, where 53% of evaluable cases had responses or stable disease. Nakagawa et al reported treating LM patients, including three having brain as the primary site, with continuous ventriculolumbar perfusion chemotherapy with some encouraging results.[86] In their study, radioiodinated ventriculography was performed to confirm the absence of obstruction to CSF flow and intracranial pressure was carefully monitored.[86] Considering the difficulty in achieving therapeutic drug levels throughout the CSF space, further attempts at ventriculolumbar perfusion would seem to be warranted, especially if less toxic therapeutic agents can be identified.

7. CONCLUSIONS

While reported relatively infrequently, LM from primary CNS tumors is a recognized and fairly well-described disease entity. Many primary CNS tumors, both malignant and benign, can lead to LM. In adults, the most common tumor to lead to LM is a high-grade glioma. Several types of pediatric brain tumors are well known to seed the neuraxis, especially medulloblastoma, ependymoma, PNET, brainstem glioma and germinoma.

While currently the incidence of LM can only be estimated, it seems that the more closely one looks, the more likely one is to find LM. Thus in the future, with improved, higher field strength MRI, it is likely that the diagnosis of LM will be made earlier and more often. Treatment for LM usually includes radiation therapy, and chemotherapy; selected surgical procedures may also be needed. Prognosis, while varying especially according to age and tumor type, is generally poor even with aggressive treatment.

Ventriculolumbar perfusion therapy and intrathecal administration of radiolabeled monoclonal antibodies have been used experimentally in patients with some intriguing results. Further information about the basic science of CNS tumor cell proliferation and metastasis is needed, and novel approaches to this disease should continue to be conceived, funded and tested.

REFERENCES

1. Ollivier, C.P. De la moelle-epinere et de ses maladies, Ed. 3. Paris, Crevat, 1837.
2. Bailey P, Cushing H. A classification of the tumors of the glioma group. Philadelphia: J.B. Lippincott Co., 1926.

3. Burger PG, Scheithauer BW, Vogel FS. Surgical Pathology of the Nervous System and Its Coverings, Fourth Ed. Philadelphia: Churchill Livingstone, pp. 160-578, 2002.
4. Maksoud YA, Hahn YS, Engelhard HH. Intracranial ependymoma. Neurosurg Focus 2002; 13:1-5.
5. Natelson SE, Dyer ML, Harp DL. Delayed CSF seeding of benign oligodendroglioma. South Med J 1992; 85:1011-2.
6. Chamberlain MC. Combined-modality treatment of leptomeningeal gliomatosis. Neurosurg 2003; 52:324-29.
7. Corsten LA, Raja AI, Wagner FC. Primary diffuse leptomeningeal gliomatosis: a case report. Brit J Neurosurg 2001; 15:62-66.
8. Dietrich PY, Aapro MS, Rieder A, Pizzolato GP. Primary diffuse leptomeningeal gliomatosis (PDLG): a neoplastic cause of chronic meningitis. J Neuro-Oncol 1993; 15:275-83.
9. Beauchesne P, Pialat J, Duthel R, et al. Aggressive treatment with complete remission in primary diffuse leptomeningeal gliomatosis – a case report. J Neuro-Oncol 1998; 37:161-7.
10. Havlik DM, Becher MW, Nolte KB. Sudden death due to primary diffuse leptomeningeal gliomatosis. J Forensic Sci 2001; 46:392-5.
11. Lachance DH, O'Neill BP, Macdonald DR, et al. Primary leptomeningeal lymphoma: report of 9 cases, diagnosis with immunohistochemical analysis, and review of the literature. Neurology 1991; 41:95-100.
12. Balhuizen JC, Bots GTAM, Schaberg A, Bosman FT. Value of cerebrospinal fluid cytology for the diagnosis of malignancies in the central nervous system. J Neurosurg 1978; 48:747-753.
13. Johnson DL, Schwarz S. Intracranial metastases from malignant spinal-cord astrocytoma. Case report. J Neurosurg 1987; 66:621-5.
14. Obana WG, Cogen PH, Davis RL, Edwards MS. Metastatic juvenile pilocytic astrocytoma. J Neurosurg 1991; 75:972-975.
15. Packer RJ, Siegel KR, Sutton LN, et al. Leptomeningeal dissemination of primary central nervous system tumors of childhood. Annals Neurol 1985; 18:217-221.
16. Nishio S, Korosue K, Tateishi J, Fukui M, Kitamura K. Ventricular and subarachnoid seeding of intracranial tumors of neuroectodermal origin – a study of 26 consecutive autopsy cases with reference to focal ependymal defect. Clin Neuropathol 1982; 1:83-91.
17. Elliott JP, Keles GE, Waite M, Temkin N, Berger MS. Ventricular entry during resection of malignant gliomas: effect on intracranial cerebrospinal fluid tumor dissemination. J Neurosurg 1994; 80:834-9.
18. Bolteus AJ, Berens ME, Pilkington GJ. Migration and invasion in brain neoplasms. Curr Neurol Neurosci Rep 2002; 1:225-32.
19. Chicoine MR, Silbergeld DL. Mitogens as motogens. J Neuro-Oncol 1997; 35:249-57.
20. Cinalli G, Sainte-Rose C, Lellouch-Tubiana A, et al. Hydrocephalus associated with intramedullary low-grade glioma. Illustrative cases and review of the literature. J Neurosurg 1995; 83:480-5.
20. Giese A, Bjerkvig R, Berens ME, Westphal M. Cost of migration: invasion of malignant gliomas and implications for treatment. J Clin Oncol 2003; 21:1624-36.
21.Binder DK, Berger MS. Proteases and the biology of glioma invasion. J Neuro-Oncol 2002; 56:149-58.
22. Engelhard HH, Narang C, Homer R, Duncan H. (1996) Urokinase antisense oligodeoxynucleotides as a novel agent for malignant glioma: *In vitro* and *in vivo* studies of uptake, effects and toxicity. Biochem Biophys Res Commun 1996; 227:400-405.
23. Levicar N, Nuttall RK, Lah TT, Nuttall RK. Proteases in brain tumor progression. Acta Neurochi 2003; 145:825-38.

24. Rooprai HK, McCormick D. Proteases and there inhibitors in human brain tumors: a review. Anticancer Res 1997; 17:4151-62.
25. Yamamoto M, Ueno Y, Hayashi S, Fukushima T. The role of proteolysis in tumor invasiveness in glioblastoma and metastatic brain tumors. Anticancer Res 2002; 22:4265-8.
26. Asano K, Kubo O, Tajika Y. et al. Expression of cadherin and CSF dissemination in malignant astrocytic tumors. Neurosurg Rev 2000; 23, 39-44.
27. Baltuch GH, Tribolet N, Van Meir EG. Expression of the CD44 adhesion molecule in tumours of the central and peripheral nervous system. J Neuro-Oncol 1995; 26:191-198.
28. Eibl RH, Pietsch T, Moll J, Skroch-Angle P. et al. Expression of varient CD44 epitopes in human astrocytic brain tumors. J Neuro-Oncol 1995; 26:165-170.
29. Kaaijk P, Troost D, Morsink F, Keehnen RMJ, et al. Expression of CD44 splice variants in human primary brain tumors. J Neuro-Oncol 1995; 26:185-190.
30. Allen JC, Epstein F. Medulloblastoma and other primary malignant neuroectodermal tumors of the CNS. J Neurosurg 1982; 57: 446-451.
31. Jennings MT, Slatkin N, D'Angelo M, et al. Neoplastic meningitis as the presentation of occult primitive neuroectodermal tumors. J Child Neurol 1993; 8:306-12.
32. Kellie SJ, Kovnar EH, Kun LE, et al. Neuraxis dissemination in pediatric brain tumors. Cancer1992; 69:1061-1066.
33. Schild SE, Nisi K, Scheithauer BW, Wong WW, Lyons MK, Schomberg PJ, Shaw EG. The results of radiotherapy for ependymomas: the Mayo Clinic experience. Intl J Radiation Oncology, Biology, Physics 1998; 42:953-8.
34. Flannery AM, Tomita T, Radkowski M, McLone DG. Medulloblastomas in childhood: postsurgical evaluation with myelography and cerebrospinal fluid cytology. J Neuro-Oncol 1990; 8: 149-51.
35. Park TS, Hoffman HJ, Hendrick EB, et al. Medulloblastoma: clinical presentation and management. J Neurosurg 1983; 58:543-552.
36. Shapiro K, Shulman, K. Spinal cord seeding from cerebellar astrocytoma. Child's Brain 1996; 2:177-186.
37. Tomita T, McLone DG. Spontaneous seeding of medulloblastoma: results of cerebrospinal fluid cytology and arachnoid biopsy from the cisterna magna. Neurosurg 1983; 12:265-7.
38. Akar Z, Tanriover N, Kafadar AM, Gazioglu N, Oz B, Kuday C. Chiasmatic low-grade glioma presenting with sacral intradural spinal metastasis. Childs Nerv Syst 2000; 16:309-11.
39. Auer RN, Rice GPA, Hinton GG, Amacher AL, Gilbert JJ Cerebellar astrocytoma with benign histology and malignant clinical course. J Neurosurg 1981; 54:128-132.
40. Civitello LA, Packer RJ, Rorke LB, Siegel K, Sutton LN, Schut L. Leptomeningeal dissemination of low-grade gliomas in children. Neurol 1988; 38:562-566.
41. Kandt RS, Shinnar S, D'Souza BJ, Singer HS, et al. Cerebrospinal metastases in malignant childhood astrocytomas. J Neuro-Oncol 1984; 2:123-128.
42. Leonard N, Alcutt DA, Farrell MA. Fatal pleomorphic xanthoastrocytoma with meningeal gliomatosis. Histopathol 1998; 32: 375-8.
43. Littmen P, Jarrett P, Bilaniuk LT, et al. Pediatric brain stem gliomas. Cancer 1980; 45:2787-2792.
44. Mishima K, Nakamura M, Nakamura H, et al. Leptomeningeal dissemination of cerebellar pilocytic astrocytoma. J Neurosurg 1992; 77:788-791.
45. Morikawa M, Tamaki N, Kokunai T, et al. Cerebellar pilocytic astrocytoma with leptomeningeal dissemination: case report. Surg Neurol 1997; 48:49-52.
46. Packer RJ, Allen J, Nielsen S, et al. Brainstem glioma: clinical manifestations of meningeal gliomatosis. Annals Neurol 1983; 14:177-182.

47. Pollack IF, Hurtt M, Pang D, Albright AL. Dissemination of low grade intracranial astrocytomas in children. Cancer1994; 73:2869-78.
48. Versari P, Talamonti G, D'Alibeti G, et al. Leptomeningeal dissemination of juvenile pilocytic astrocytoma: case report. Surg Neurol 1994; 41:318-321.
49. Aoyama I, Makita, Y, Nabeshima S, Moomochi M, Masuda A. Extradural nasal and orbital extension of glioblastoma multiforme without previous surgical intervention. Surg Neurol 1980; 14:343-7.
50. Awad I, Bay JW, Rogers L. Leptomeningeal metastasis from supratentorial malignant gliomas. Neurosurgery 1986; 19:247-251.
51. Coakham HB, Richardson RB, Davies AG, Bourne SP, Eckert H, Kemshead JT. Neoplastic meningitis from a pineal tumor treated by antibody-guided irradiation via the intrathecal route. British J Neurosurg 1988; 2:199-209.
52. Eng DY, DeMonte F, Ginsberg L, Fuller GN, Jaeckle K. Craniospinal dissemination of central neurocytoma. Report of two cases. J Neurosurg 1997; 86:547-52.
53. Gajjar A, Bhargava R, Jenkins JJ. Low-grade astrocytoma with neuraxis dissemination at diagnosis. J Neurosurg 1995; 83:67-71.
54. Gaspar LE, Mackenzie IR, Gilbert JJ, et al. Primary cerebral fibrosarcomas. Clinicopathologic study and review of the literature. Cancer 1993; 72:3277-81.
55. Giordana MT, Cavalla P, Allegranza A, Pollo B. Intracranial dissemination of pituitary adenoma. Case report and review of the literature. Italian J Neurolog Sci 1994; 15:195-200.
56. Grossman SA, Celano P. Neoplastic meningitis. N Engl J Med 2001; 344:494.
57. Ito M, Jamshidi J, Yamanaka K. Does craniopharyngioma metastasize? Case report and review of the literature. Neurosurg 2001; 48:933-5.
58. Kamiya K, Inagawa T, Nagasako R. Malignant intraventricular meningioma with spinal metastasis through the cerebrospinal fluid. Surg Neurol 1989; 32:213-8.
59. Kawano N, Yada K, Ogawa Y, Sasaki K. Spontaneous transdural extension of malignant astrocytoma. J Neurosurg 1977; 47:766-770.
60. Kim JH, Jung HW, Kim YS, et al. Meningeal hemangiopericytomas: long term outcome and biological behavior. Surg Neurol 2003; 59:47-53.
61. Ley A, Campillo D, Oliveras C. Extracranial metastasis of glioblastoma multiforme. J Neurosurg 1961; 18:313-330.
62. Mantravadi RVP, Phatak R, Bellur S, et al. Brainstem gliomas: an autopsy study of 25 cases. Cancer1982; 49:1294-1296.
63. Moore MT, Eisinger G. Extra primary seeding of glioblastoma multiforme in the subarachnoid space and ependyma. Neurol 1963; 13: 855-865.
64. Ng HK, Tang NL, Poon WS. Polar spongioblastoma with cerebrospinal fluid metastases. Surg Neurol 1994; 41:137-42.
65. Silverberg GD, Hanbery JW. Meningeal invasion by gliomas. J Neurosurg 1971; 34:549-554.
66. Tognetti F, Piazza G, Morrone B. High grade astrocytoma with spontaneous meningeal and cranial invasion. Neurosurg 1982; 11:813-815.
67. Wai-kwan AY, Horten BC, Shapiro WR. Meningeal gliomatosis: a review of 12 cases. Ann Neurol 1980; 8:605-608.
68. Yamaki T, Otaki M, Uede T, et al. Extensive spinal necrosis with spinal leptomeningeal dissemination of cerebral astrocytoma: case report. Acta Neurochir 1988; 93:146-148.
69. Bell WO, Packer RJ, Seigel KR, Borke, LB, Sutton, LN, Bruce, D.A., Schut, L. Leptomeningeal spread of intramedullary spinal cord tumors. J Neurosurg 1988; 69:295-300.
71. Hely M, Fryer J, Selby G. Intramedullary spinal cord glioma with intracranial seeding. J Neurol Neurosurg Psych 1985; 48:302-9.

72. Ng HK, Leung CH, Boet R, Poon WS. Spinal cord pilocytic astrocytoma with cranial meningeal metastases. J Clin Neuroscience 2001; 8:374-7.
73. Erlich SS, Davis RL. Spinal subarachnoid metastases from primary intracranial glioblastoma multiforme. Cancer 1978; 42:2854-64.
74. Onda K, Tanaka R, Takahashi H, Takeda N, Ikuta F. Cerebral glioblastoma with cerebrospinal fluid dissemination: a clinicopathological study of 14 cases examined by complete autopsy. Neurosurg 1989; 25:533-40.
75. Engelhard HH, Porter KR, Stewart AK, Olson JJ. Overview of the results of the Commission on Cancer's Central Nervous System (CNS) Tumor Patient Care Evaluation Study. Proc Am Assoc Cancer Res 2004; 45:164.
76. Murakami M, Kuratsu J, Takeshima H, et al. Spinal seeding of anaplastic ependymoma mimicking fungal meningitis. A case report and review of the literature. J Neurosurg Sci 2000; 44:46-51.
77. Trivedi RA, Nichols P, Coley S, et al. Leptomeningeal glioblastoma presenting with multiple cranial neuropathies and confusion. Clin Neurol Neurosurg 2000; 102:223-6.
78. Fujimura M, Kumabe T, Jokura H, Shirane R, Yoshimoto T, Tominaga T. Intractable vomiting as an early clinical symptom of cerebrospinal fluid seeding to the fourth ventricle in patients with high-grade astrocytoma. J Neuro-Oncol 2004; 66:209-16.
79. Tamura, Zama A, Kurihara H, et al. Management of recurrent pilocytic astrocytoma with leptomeningeal dissemination in childhood. Childs Nerv Syst 1998; 14:617-22.
80. Packer RJ, Sutton LN, Rorke LB, et al. Prognostic importance of cellular differentiation in medulloblastoma of childhood. J Neurosurg 1984; 61:296-301.
81. Black PM, Callahan LV, Kornblith PL. Tissue cultures from cerebrospinal fluid specimens in the study of human brain tumors. J Neurosurg 1978; 49:697-704.
82. Witham TF, Fukui MB, Meltzer CC, et al. Survival of patients with high grade glioma treated with intrathecal thiotriethylenephosphoramide for ependymal or leptomeningeal gliomatosis. Cancer 1999; 86:1347-53.
83. Engelhard HH, Misra M, Rosen FR. Interstitial chemotherapy for the treatment of malignant glioma. Adv Clin Neurosci 2000; 10:341-53.
84. Engelhard HH, Petruska DA. Movement and imaging of iron oxide- bound antibodies in brain and cerebrospinal fluid. Cancer Biochem Biophys 1992; 13:224-36.
85. Coakham HB, Kemshead JT. Treatment of neoplastic meningitis by targeted radiation using (131)I-radiolabelled monoclonal antibodies. Results of responses and long term follow-up in 40 patients. J Neuro-Oncol 1998; 38:225-32.
86. Nakagawa H, Fujita T, Kubo S, et al. Ventriculolumbar perfusion chemotherapy with methotrexate and cytosine arabinoside for meningeal carcinomatosis: a pilot study in 13 patients. Surg Neurol 1996; 45:256-64.

Chapter 6

LEPTOMENINGEAL CANCER IN THE PEDIATRIC PATIENT

Kathleen A. Neville, M.D, and Susan M. Blaney, M.D
Texas Children's Cancer Center, Baylor College of Medicine
Houston, TX 77030

Abstract: The treatment and prophylaxis of leptomeningeal leukemia and lymphoma in children has dramatically improved disease control and long-term survival. However, the treatment of other leptomeningeal cancers has been less successful and the neurologic morbidity associated with central nervous system-directed therapy has a significant long-term impact on quality of life. Further research is critical to identify new therapeutic strategies for children with or at high risk for leptomeningeal cancer.

Key words: Acute lymphoblastic leukemia; neuroblastoma; craniospinal irradiation; prophylactic intrathecal therapy; medulloblastoma

1. INTRODUCTION

Leptomeningeal dissemination of pediatric tumors occurs most frequently in children who have leukemia or a primary central nervous system (CNS) tumor; however, it may also be observed in a variety of other solid tumors of childhood. The initial recognition that the CNS serves as a sanctuary site, protected from the effects of most systemically administered chemotherapy, occurred more than 30 years ago in children with acute lymphoblastic leukemia.[1,2] The high incidence of CNS leukemic relapse following the introduction of effective systemic combination chemotherapy for bone marrow disease highlighted the limitations imposed by the blood-brain barrier. The incorporation of specific CNS-targeted therapeutic strategies, including radiation therapy and intrathecal drug delivery, into the frontline treatment of childhood leukemia resulted in a great advance in the prevention and treatment of leptomeningeal leukemia in this patient. Unfortunately, although tremendous strides have been made in the treatment and prevention of leptomeningeal leukemia, this success has not yet been realized in either the treatment or the prevention of most other leptomeningeal cancers of childhood. In this chapter, we will summarize the current status of the recognition, diagnosis, and management of childhood cancers that have a predilection for leptomeningeal dissemination.

2. CLINICAL PRESENTATION OF CHILDREN WITH LEPTOMENINGEAL METASTASES

The signs and symptoms of leptomeningeal dissemination are highly variable depending upon the extent and location of the disease. Although symptoms may be focal, it is important to remember that leptomeningeal metastases affect the entire neuraxis, necessitating evaluation and treatment of the brain and spinal cord. Children with an underlying primary CNS or solid tumor are more likely to have leptomeningeal dissemination in association with advanced systemic or bulky CNS disease than children with underlying leukemias or lymphomas. As a result, there are myriad signs and symptoms, related to either the primary tumor or to leptomeningeal spread of the tumor, that may be present at initial diagnosis. In contrast, some children with leptomeningeal metastases may be relatively asymptomatic at initial diagnosis, particularly if the diagnosis occurs in association with periodic surveillance laboratory (e.g., cerebrospinal fluid (CSF) cytology) or neuroimaging studies.

Signs and symptoms of leptomeningeal dissemination are dependent on the site(s) of neuraxis involvement.[3-9] The most common signs and symptoms are a result of increased intracranial pressure and include headache, nausea, and vomiting. Cranial nerve involvement may result in double vision, loss of hearing, loss of vision, or facial numbness and weakness. Signs and symptoms due to spinal cord involvement may include weakness, sensory loss, pain, numbness, ataxia, or paraparesis. With leptomeningeal disease progression, children may develop confusion, memory loss, dementia, seizures, or mental status changes.

3. DIAGNOSIS OF LEPTOMENINGEAL METASTASES IN CHILDHOOD CANCER

The diagnosis of leptomeningeal metastases is primarily based on results of CSF and neuroimaging studies. Evaluation of the CSF remains the single most important diagnostic tool in patients with an underlying leukemia or lymphoma. With the routine use of gadolinium-enhanced magnetic resonance imaging (MRI), neuroradiographic studies have played an increasingly important role in the diagnosis of leptomeningeal metastases in patients with underlying CNS or solid tumors.

3.1 Cerebrospinal fluid studies

Essential elements in the laboratory evaluation of CSF include cell count, cytology and determination of CSF protein and glucose concentrations. There is no single CSF biochemical marker or CSF laboratory test that is diagnostic of leptomeningeal tumor spread. In children with underlying CNS or solid tumors, the presence of malignant cells in the CSF is diagnostic of leptomeningeal metastases. However, a negative CSF cytology result does not preclude the diagnosis of leptomeningeal metastases. Studies in adults with leptomeningeal disease have demonstrated that initial CSF cytology samples are positive in only 55-70% of patients but, with repeated CSF sampling, the incidence of positive cytology increases to 80-92%.[4,10] Thus, serial examination of CSF, including sampling from alternate sites (e.g. ventricular or cisternal) may be required for the detection of malignant cells. However, despite repeated CSF sampling some children will have persistently negative CSF cytology. In such patients, the presence of appropriate neuroimaging abnormalities is adequate for the diagnosis of leptomeningeal metastasis.[11]

There is some controversy about the objective definition of overt CNS leukemia. Traditionally, the diagnosis of CNS leukemia required the presence of greater than 5 CSF leukocytes/μL plus the presence of lymphoblasts on a CSF cytospin. However, several retrospective studies have demonstrated that the presence of any CSF lymphoblasts placed patients at higher risk of subsequent leptomeningeal relapse even if there were fewer than 5 leukocytes/μL;[12,13] other studies, however, failed to confirm these findings.[14] Therefore, in an attempt to clarify the significance of positive CSF cytology despite a low CSF leukocyte count, some current frontline chemotherapy trials have developed a separate treatment stratum, CNS-2 (Table 1) in which children who have fewer than 5 leukocytes/μL and lymphoblasts receive a more intensive CNS-directed therapy than patients with fewer than 5 leukocytes/μL and no lymphoblasts; however, it is less intensive in those with greater than 5 leukocytes/μL and lymphoblasts.

Table 1. Classification of CNS Disease Status in Patients with Leukemia Based on CSF Findings at Initial Diagnosis

Status	CSF Findings
CNS-1	No lymphoblasts
CNS-2	< 5 WBCs/μL with definable blasts on cytocentrifuge examination
CNS-3	≥5 WBCs/μL with blast cells (or cranial nerve palsy)

In some cases of CNS leukemia or lymphoma, it may be difficult to confirm the diagnosis because lymphocytes in the CSF are not always readily identifiable as malignant by the cytopathologist. In such instances, abnormal CSF cytogenetic or flow cytometry results may further support the diagnosis. In children who have germ cell tumors, elevations in tumor markers such as α-fetoprotein (AFP) or the β-subunit of human chorionic gonadotropin (HCG) may support the diagnosis of leptomeningeal metastases. Elevations in AFP are more common in the non-germinomatous germ cell tumors, whereas elevations in β-HCG are more common in choriocarcinomas and some germinomas.[15] When evaluating tumor marker levels, it is important to simultaneously assess serum and CSF in order to ascertain whether or not an elevated marker is the result of passive diffusion into the CSF or secondary to leptomeningeal dissemination.[16]

Other non-specific abnormalities that are frequently found in the CSF of patients with leptomeningeal metastases include an elevated opening pressure, a decrease in glucose concentration, and an increase in protein concentration. Since some children with primary CNS tumors have indwelling ventriculoperitoneal shunts, it is important to remember that the lumbar CSF protein level may be increased in the absence of leptomeningeal metastases due to shunt-induced alterations in CSF flow. In addition, in children with leptomeningeal metastases who have indwelling Ommaya reservoirs, CSF studies for staging and diagnosis must include an evaluation of both ventricular and lumbar CSF spaces since lumbar CSF cytology is frequently positive in the presence of negative ventricular CSF cytology.[17]

3.2 Neuroimaging studies

Neuroimaging studies are extremely useful in defining the extent of leptomeningeal disease in children who have underlying primary CNS or solid tumors. Neuroimaging studies also facilitate the identification of areas of bulky disease and the assessment of CSF flow dynamics. In children with CNS leukemia, neuroimaging studies of the brain and/or spinal cord are sometimes obtained if there are focal neurological symptoms (e.g. cranial nerve palsies, visual problems, or localized pain). Furthermore, it is not unreasonable to obtain a baseline head MRI at the initial diagnosis of CNS leukemia or lymphoma.

As with CSF cytology, negative imaging studies do not preclude a diagnosis of leptomeningeal metastases. It has been suggested that if there is a strong clinical suspicion of neoplastic meningitis in the presence of negative cytology and neuroimaging studies, that obtaining a high-dose gadolinium-enhanced MRI may increase the diagnostic yield.[18]

3.3 CSF flow studies

Nuclear medicine CSF flow studies (^{111}indium-diethylenetriamine pentaacetic acid (DTPA) or technetium Tc^{99}-DTPA) should be performed in children with non-leukemic leptomeningeal metastases prior to the administration of intrathecal chemotherapy. CSF flow studies provide a dynamic evaluation of the functional anatomy of the various CSF compartments and can detect flow abnormalities that may not be apparent on conventional neuroradiographic imaging.[5,6] Obstruction of the normal circulation of CSF flow by tumor may lead to either decreased drug efficacy due to inadequate distribution throughout the neuraxis or increased toxicity because of high local drug concentrations.

Abnormalities in CSF flow, observed in approximately one-third of adults with leptomeningeal metastases, appear to adversely affect the response to treatment and overall prognosis.[19,20] Prospective studies correlating the results of CSF flow studies and response to treatment or prognosis have not been performed in children. However, the overall incidence of abnormalities in CSF flow in children with leptomeningeal metastases at diagnosis appears to be lower than in adults. This probably reflects the fact that the initial diagnosis of leptomeningeal dissemination in many children is temporally associated with surveillance MRIs or CSF cytology studies, i.e. at a time when patients may be relatively less symptomatic or even asymptomatic.

4. CHILDHOOD TUMORS WITH A PREDILECTION FOR LEPTOMENINGEAL DISSEMINATION

4.1 Leukemias/Lymphoma

Prior to the institution of prophylactic, or "pre-symptomatic" CNS therapy, CNS leukemia occurred in more than 50% of children with acute lymphoblastic leukemia (ALL) and was a major cause of treatment failure in patients who achieved bone marrow remission.[1,2] However, with the incorporation of effective CNS prophylaxis into frontline treatment, leptomeningeal leukemia is now a relatively uncommon event occurring in fewer than 10% of patients.[21] Standard pre-symptomatic therapy for all children with leukemia includes intrathecal chemotherapy with methotrexate administered as a single agent or in combination with cytarabine and dexamethasone. Children who are at high risk of CNS recurrence may also receive prophylactic cranial radiation.

4.1.1 Treatment

In the past, the long-term outcome for children with an isolated CNS relapse was dismal because a bone marrow relapse invariably followed. However, current treatment approaches that include intrathecal chemotherapy plus intensive systemic chemotherapy, followed by delayed consolidation with craniospinal irradiation (CSI), and maintenance therapy with intrathecal and systemic chemotherapy, have dramatically improved the long-term outlook for children with an initial isolated CNS relapse who have not previously received CSI. Results of a recent Pediatric Oncology Group (POG) study evaluating the efficacy of delaying radiation therapy for six months after an isolated CNS relapse demonstrated a 4-year event free survival of 71% ± 5% for all patients, an event free survival of 83% ± 5.3% for children whose relapse occurred more than 18 months after initial diagnosis and 46.2 ± 10.2% for those with a first complete remission of less than 18 months.[22,23] The rationale for delaying CSI in patients with an overt CNS relapse is to allow delivery of early intensive systemic chemotherapy in an attempt to prevent a subsequent bone marrow relapse. Current clinical trials for children with an isolated CNS relapse are evaluating the feasibility of delaying radiation for 12 months as well as delivering cranial radiation only, rather than CSI, if the initial relapse is greater than 18 months after initial diagnosis.

The long-term prognosis is poor for children who experience a CNS leukemic relapse after definitive irradiation to the neuraxis. Although the optimal treatment regimen for a second or greater CNS relapse has not been defined, both systemic and CNS-directed therapy is required. In general, treatment decisions should be guided by prior systemic and CNS-directed therapy. CNS-directed treatment approaches for such patients include intrathecal administration of standard agents via an Ommaya reservoir or administration of new intrathecal agents undergoing evaluation in the phase I or phase II setting.

Intrathecal chemotherapy using a "concentration times time" ("CxT") approach via an indwelling ventricular access device has been successful in inducing CNS remissions even in patients who have a CNS recurrence while receiving standard dose intralumbar therapy. The "C x T" schedule consists of repeated intraventricular administration of low-dose chemotherapy (methotrexate alternated with cytarabine) over a relatively short period of time. This delivery schedule increases the duration of CSF exposure to cytotoxic drug concentrations, which is critical for cell-cycle specific agents such as methotrexate and cytarabine. It may also lessen the incidence of neurotoxicity by avoiding high peak drug concentrations and deliver of a lower cumulative drug dose over time.[24]

Development of sustained release agents for intrathecal administration represents an extension of the "CxT" approach. A sustained release formulation of liposomal cytarabine (DepoCyt™), recently approved by the Food and Drug Administration for treatment of lymphomatous meningitis in adults, has a terminal half-life that is 40-fold greater than the standard intrathecal cytarabine (141 h vs 3.4 h).[25,26] A Phase I trial of liposomal cytarabine in children with refractory or recurrent leptomeningeal cancers is nearing completion.[27] Future studies will define the role of this agent in the treatment of childhood CNS leukemia.

The role of bone marrow transplantation in the treatment of a CNS leukemic relapse is not known and there are inadequate patient numbers to compare this approach prospectively to other traditional approaches. Nevertheless, there are anecdotal reports indicating that transplant can induce prolonged disease- free survival in some patients with a history of CNS disease. However, such patients are at increased risk of treatment-related toxicity, especially CNS complications.[28]

Although leptomeningeal dissemination of lymphoma is unusual at initial presentation, it appears to be more common in patients who have bone marrow disease.[29] Similar to leukemias, lymphomatous meningitis will eventually occur in a high proportion of patients if presymptomatic therapy is not incorporated into front-line treatment. In addition to leptomeningeal spread, CNS involvement from lymphoma can also include cranial nerve infiltration, parenchymal CNS disease, paraspinal tumor or a combination of these.[29] CNS involvement appears to be most common in patients with African Burkitt's lymphoma.[29] The approach to the treatment of children with recurrent or refractory leptomeningeal lymphoma is similar to that for children who have CNS leukemia.

5. PRIMARY CNS TUMORS

Leptomeningeal dissemination may occur in a wide variety of childhood brain tumors including medulloblastoma, supratentorial primitive neuroectodermal tumor (PNET), atypical teratoid/rhabdoid tumor (ATRT), glioma, ependymoma and germ cell tumors.[3,15,30-38] Dissemination may be present at initial diagnosis, occur in combination with local disease progression or relapse, or occur as an isolated event. Younger children appear to be at higher risk for leptomeningeal spread. The reported incidence of leptomeningeal dissemination for a given histologic tumor subtype often varies widely from series to series. In the past, staging of the entire neuraxis was not routinely performed. However, the widespread availability of gadolinium-enhanced MRIs has facilitated routine neuraxis staging for the majority of children with a newly diagnosed CNS tumor. Other factors that may influence the variability between reports is underlying referral patterns to various children's hospitals or treatment centers.

5.1 Medulloblastoma (Infratentorial Primitive Neuroectodermal Tumors)

Medulloblastoma has a great propensity for leptomeningeal dissemination relative to other pediatric CNS tumors. Leptomeningeal metastases are present at diagnosis in up to 27-43% of infants and young children with medulloblastoma, compared with an incidence of less than 20-25% in older children with similar histologic diagnosis.[15] The reported incidence of leptomeningeal spread is greater than 90% in patients with medulloblastoma who come to autopsy.[15,39,40]

Because of the predilection for leptomeningeal dissemination, CSI is an integral component of therapy for all children with newly diagnosed medulloblastoma who are over three years of age. Results of recent pediatric cooperative group studies, including a trial that compared conventional dose radiation (36 Gy to the neuraxis and 54 Gy to the posterior fossa) versus reduced dose radiation (25 Gy to the neuraxis and 54 Gy to the posterior fossa suggest that post-surgical treatment with reduced-dose CSI therapy and adjuvant chemotherapy does not adversely impact event-free survival and may improve neuropsychological outcome in patients who do not have overt leptomeningeal disease.[41-43]

CSI followed by adjuvant chemotherapy is also a successful treatment strategy for the majority of children who have leptomeningeal metastases at initial diagnosis.[44] However, children who experience a leptomeningeal relapse during or after completion of standard therapy have a dismal prognosis. Leptomeningeal medulloblastoma is usually rapidly progressive and there is no known curative therapy. Some children have experienced transient benefit after palliative treatment with oral etoposide[45,46] or treatment with investigational intrathecal agents such as mafosfamide or topotecan.[27] There is currently a Phase II Children's Oncology Group study to evaluate the response rate and progression-free survival for children with leptomeningeal medulloblastoma treated with intrathecal topotecan.

The optimal treatment for children $\leq$3 years with PNET/medulloblastoma remains unknown since CSI in young children and infants is associated with an unacceptably high incidence of neuropsychologic and neuroendocrine sequelae. Recent treatment strategies for this age group have focused on the delivery of post-operative chemotherapy in an attempt to delay the need for neuraxis radiation. Unfortunately, these efforts have had a limited impact since most infants have either a local or disseminated disease recurrence within six to nine months of initial diagnosis.[47-50] Infants who progress while receiving their initial chemotherapy can be salvaged with CSI. However, all infants treated in this fashion have a substantial decline or loss in cognitive function and most experience neuroendocrine problems.[51] Therefore, in an attempt to control leptomeningeal disease without the morbidity associated with neuraxis irradiation to the developing CNS, the Pediatric Brain Tumor Consortium is currently evaluating a treatment strategy that utilizes up-front systemic chemotherapy plus intrathecal chemotherapy and the early introduction of limited-field conformal radiation therapy.

5.2 Supratentorial PNETs

Supratentorial PNETs occur predominately in the cerebral hemispheres. The incidence of leptomeningeal dissemination for supratentorial PNETs varies markedly between series. However, it appears that the overall incidence at initial presentation is lower in children with medulloblastoma, ranging from 5 - 10%. Nevertheless, CSI is recommended as a component of the initial treatment for children with supratentorial PNETs because the eventual occurrence of leptomeningeal spread may be as high as 70%.[15]

5.3 Ependymomas

The reported incidence of leptomeningeal dissemination in children with ependymomas ranges from 3% - 22%.[15,52] Until recently, there was ongoing debate about the need for prophylactic CSI in the absence of leptomeningeal dissemination. At the present time, most investigators limit the use of CSI in ependymoma to children with objective evidence of leptomeningeal spread.[52] In a recent retrospective series neither evidence for dissemination at presentation nor the detection of anaplastic histological features were associated with a significantly worse outcome.[52] Age of the patient at diagnosis, and extent of surgical resection, appear to be the most important prognostic factors in the initial treatment of this disease.[15,52]

5.4 Gliomas

Low-grade gliomas have an approximately 3%-4% incidence of leptomeningeal spread;[34] while higher grade supratentorial and brainstem gliomas have a higher incidence of spread, ranging from 20-45% across various retrospective series.[33,35,53,54] Disseminated disease due to pilocytic or other low grade astrocytomas does not necessarily preclude long-term survival since such tumors rarely show malignant degeneration;[55] long-term survival has been reported following treatment with CSI.[54,56-60] In contrast, the median survival after the diagnosis of leptomeningeal dissemination from anaplastic gliomas is three to four months. [35,38]

Diffuse leptomeningeal gliomatosis, a condition characterized by glioma in the leptomeninges without a primary mass lesion in the CNS,[61] is rare in adults and extremely rare in children. The diagnosis is often difficult to distinguish from subacute meningitis of multiple infectious or non-infectious etiologies [62,63]. Clinically, patients may present with a prodromal phase of generalized malaise followed by rapid neurologic deterioration.[64] In general, the prognosis for children with leptomeningeal gliomatosis is dismal, although some patients may experience transient benefit from radiation and chemotherapy. [61,65]

5.5 Pineal-area tumors

Pineal masses, uncommon in pediatric patients, may include pineoblastomas, germ cell tumors, and astrocytomas. The overall incidence of leptomeningeal spread for children with non-astrocytic pineal-area tumors, including pineoblastoma and germinoma, is approximately 10% at initial diagnosis.[15,66] CSI is the standard therapy for non-germinomatous germ cell tumors (embryonal carcinoma, endodermal sinus tumor, or choriocarcinoma), pineoblastomas, and germinomas with evidence of leptomeningeal dissemination. The role of chemotherapy on the long-term outcome of patients with pineal-area tumors is not clear because of their relative rarity. However, there are chemotherapy regimens, including platinum plus etoposide, or cyclophosphamide, that may facilitate delivery of reduced dose CSI for children with CNS germ cell tumors, including those with leptomeningeal spread at initial diagnosis.[67,68]

5.6 Choroid plexus tumors

Choroid plexus tumors, including choroid plexus carcinoma and choroid plexus papilloma, account for 1-3% of all pediatric brain tumors; generally present during the first two years life.[69-71] Extensive disease, including leptomeningeal metastases, has been reported in up to 70% of infants with choroid plexus carcinoma. Multi-modality therapy with surgery, chemotherapy, and radiation has been effective for some patients. The efficacy of adjuvant therapy in terms of both chemotherapy and radiotherapy remains unclear due to limited data.[69] However, it appears that CSI is a required component of therapy for patients with metastatic disease or a subtotal resection. [69]

5.7 Meningioma

Although meningiomas are a common primary CNS tumor in adults, they are rare in children representing less than 2% of all pediatric CNS tumors.[72] Unfortunately, the prognosis in children is comparatively poor due to rapid growth, malignant change, and likely recurrence.[73-77] Although meningiomas primarily present with bulky disease, leptomeningeal metastases can occur.[78,79] Clear-cell meningioma, a rare and more aggressive subtype,[80] appears to have a particular propensity for diffuse leptomeningeal seeding.[81]

6. SOLID TUMORS

Leptomeningeal metastases may also occur in a variety of childhood solid tumors including retinoblastoma,[82] neuroblastoma,[83-86] rhabdomyosarcoma,[87] melanoma,[88,89] and Ewing's sarcoma.[90,91] These metastases occur most commonly when advanced systemic disease is present, either at the time of initial diagnosis or when the primary tumor has recurred.

6.1 Rhabdomyosarcoma

Rhabdomyosarcoma can invade the base of the skull and extend intracranially with subsequent leptomeningeal metastases. The four anatomic sites with the potential for leptomeningeal spread are the nasopharynx/nasal cavity, the middle ear, the paranasal sinuses, and the infratemporal fossa/pterygopalatine space.[92] These sites comprise approximately 15% of all rhabdomyosarcomas. In the past, treatment for rhabdomyosarcoma involving these sites included whole brain radiotherapy. However, over the past several decades, radiation ports have gradually been refined to eliminate the need for cranial radiotherapy.[92] Current practice for lesions at high risk for leptomeningeal spread is radiation therapy to refined ports with 1.5 cm margins around the gross tumor volume.

6.2 Retinoblastoma

Leptomeningeal spread of retinoblastoma is believed to occur via direct propagation from the retina along the optic nerve to the chiasm and leptomeninges.[93] It may also occur via extension from the choroid into the meningeal spaces,[94] or along the central retinal vessels to the subarachnoid space. [95] The prognosis for patients with meningeal metastases is invariably poor regardless of the chemotherapy regimen;[82] death from metastatic disease occurs an average of five to six months from onset. [96]

6.3 Neuroblastoma

Parenchymal and/or leptomeningeal dissemination in children with metastatic neuroblastoma is relatively uncommon, occurring in approximately 5% of children with Stage IV disease.[83-86,97] In fact, the CNS may be the first or only site of progressive disease.[83] Recent retrospective reviews suggest that as treatment for the underlying systemic neuroblastoma improves, the incidence of CNS neuroblastoma may be increasing.[97] Clinically, leptomeningeal dissemination of neuroblastoma is progressive.

6.4 Ewing's Sarcoma

Although leptomeningeal dissemination has been reported in children who have Ewing's sarcoma, it is uncommon occurring in less than 3% of patients.[90,98] Leptomeningeal metastases are generally observed in children who have advanced systemic disease rather than as an isolated event. [91,98] Prophylactic treatment of the CNS with cranial radiation and/or intrathecal therapy is not warranted due to the low overall incidence of CNS spread; historically, CNS prophylaxis has not prevented subsequent leptomeningeal spread. [87]

6.5 Melanoma

Melanoma is one of the most common leptomeningeal cancers in adults; however, it is infrequently observed in children since melanoma comprises less than 1% of childhood cancers.[88,99] Leptomeningeal dissemination of melanoma most commonly occurs in children who have advanced systemic disease, especially underlying CNS parenchymal metastases. Children who have large congenital nevi rarely present with primary leptomeningeal melanoma.[88,99] Both primary leptomeningeal melanoma and metastatic leptomeningeal melanoma are rapidly progressive entities for which there is no known effective therapy. In contrast, neurocutaneous melanosis (NCM), a rare phacomatosis characterized by the presence of large non-malignant melanocytic nevi in combination with an excess of melanotic cells in the leptomeninges may be asymptomatic for prolonged periods or have neurologic symptoms with or without associated malignant transformation. The prognosis for patients with neurologic symptoms is generally poor, even in the absence of malignant involvement. [88,100-102]

7. TREATMENT OF LEPTOMENINGEAL METASTASES

The optimal treatment for tumors with a predilection for leptomeningeal metastases is preventative or presymptomatic therapy. This approach has been successfully employed for the vast majority of children with leukemias or lymphomas and, to a somewhat lesser extent, for medulloblastoma or supratentorial PNET through utilization of CNS-targeted treatment approaches with intrathecal chemotherapy or CSI. CNS-directed treatment approaches have also been increasingly successful in the treatment of initial isolated CNS leukemic relapses as well for some CNS tumors with leptomeningeal metastases at diagnosis, including medulloblastoma and low- grade gliomas. Unfortunately, for the majority of children who have refractory CNS leukemia, leptomeningeal medulloblastoma after neuraxis radiation, or leptomeningeal metastases from most other underlying solid or CNS tumors, the outlook is dismal with rapid progression over a period of weeks to months. The remainder of this section will focus on treatment considerations for these latter patients with high-risk, poor prognosis disease.

The initial evaluation of a child with high risk, poor prognosis leptomeningeal metastases requires a thorough initial assessment of symptoms or neurologic deficits that may be palliated that may be preserved with early therapeutic intervention(s). Examples of such signs and symptoms include headache, pain, cranial nerve palsies, visual loss, weakness, or loss of neurologic function. Treatment with analgesics, steroids, and/or focal radiation therapy to areas of bulk disease should be considered. Patients with acute loss of function are more likely to be completely or partially restored with a therapeutic intervention than those with sub-acute or chronic deficits. Interventions for acute or rapidly progressive lesions must occur as expeditiously as possible in order to maximize improved or restored function.

The extent of leptomeningeal metastases, as well as the status of the primary underlying malignancy, must also be defined. This information, coupled with an assessment of the performance status and rate of disease progression, serves as a guide in evaluating whether or not the patient is a candidate for enrollment in ongoing clinical trials. In general, children who have advanced disease and a poor performance status are offered symptomatic or palliative therapy; children who have an adequate performance status and less advanced disease should be considered as potential candidates for ongoing phase I or phase II clinical trials.

The decision to treat with a systemic or intrathecal agent should be guided in part by a knowledge of the extent of the leptomeningeal metastases. Children with extensive and "bulky" leptomeningeal disease are less likely to benefit from an intrathecal approach than children with positive cytology or minimal leptomeningeal enhancement, due to the limited tissue penetration (~ 3-4 mm) of intrathecally administered chemotherapy.[103] In addition, as previously discussed, extensive leptomeningeal disease may also cause alterations in CSF flow (e.g. obstruction) that may preclude intrathecal drug administration.[104] For such patients, it may therefore be preferable to pursue systemic chemotherapy, preferably with an agent that penetrates the blood-CSF barrier.

Agents for intrathecal administration that are currently being evaluated in phase I and phase II clinical trials include topotecan, a topoisomerase I poison; mafosfamide, a pre-activated analog of cyclophosphamide; liposomal cytarabine, a sustained release formulation of cytarabine, and busulfan, an alkylating agent. The role of these agents in the treatment of leptomeningeal metastases in childhood cancer has not yet been defined.

7.1 Treatment sequelae

The nervous system is exquisitely sensitive to the potential adverse sequelae of CNS-directed therapy. For example, intrathecal therapy may be associated with acute, sub-acute or chronic toxicities including paralysis and leukoencephalopathy.[105,106] Likewise, radiation therapy may be associated with significant adverse effects including neuroendocrine deficits, neuropsychological deficits, leukoencephalopathy, and second malignancies.[107-114] In addition to the toxicities associated with each specific agent or modality of therapy, there are many other variables that may affect the incidence and toxicities associated with CNS-directed therapy. These include the age at the time of therapy, concomitantly administered systemic therapies (e.g. methotrexate), and cumulative dose of specific therapeutic agents.[115]

8. CONCLUSION

Leptomeningeal cancer remains a challenging problem for pediatric oncologists. Despite considerable progress in the treatment and prevention of leptomeningeal cancer due to leukemias and lymphomas, the long-term outcome for children with leptomeningeal disease due to brain tumors and other solid tumors remains poor. In addition, there are significant toxicities associated with CNS-directed therapy in those children who are ultimately cured. Further research is clearly needed to identify new agents and treatment strategies for children with, or at high risk of developing leptomeningeal metastases. These efforts must be focused not only at the identification of effective treatments or treatment strategies, but also at the identification of approaches that are associated with minimal potential for neurotoxicity.

REFERENCES

1. Evans A, Gilbert E, Zandstra R. The increasing incidence of central nervous system leukemia in children. Cancer 1970; 26:404-407.
2. Hardisty R, Norman P. Meningeal leukemia. Arch Dis Child 1967; 42:441-447.
3. Bleyer W, Byrne T. Leptomeningeal cancer in leukemia and solid tumors. Curr Probl Cancer 1988; 4:185-238.
4. Wasserstrom W, Glass J, Posner J. Diagnosis and treatment of leptomeningeal metastases from solid tumors: experience with 90 patients. Cancer 1982; 49:759-772.
5. Chamberlain M, Kormanik P. Prognostic significance of 111indium-DTPA CSF flow studies in leptomeningeal metastases. Neurology 1996; 46:1674-1677.
6. Chamberlain M, Corey-Bloom J. Leptomeningeal metastases: 111 indium-DTPA CSF flow studies. Neurology 1991; 41:1765-1769.
7. Little J, Dale A, Okazaki H. Meningeal carcinomatosis. Arch Neurol 1974;30:138-143.
8. Olson M, Chernik N, Posner J. Infiltration of the leptomeninges by systemic cancer. A clinical and pathologic study. Arch Neurol 1974;30:122-137.
9. Theodore W, Gendelman S. Meningeal carcinomatosis. Arch Neurol 1981;38:696-699.
10. Kaplan J, DeSouza T, Farkash A, et al. Leptomeningeal metastases: comparison of clinical 0features and laboratory data of solid tumors, lymphomas, and leukemias. J Neurooncol. 1990; 9:225-229.
11. Freilich R, Krol G, DeAngelis L. Neuroimaging and cerebrospinal fluid cytology in the diagnosis of leptomeningeal metastasis. Ann Neurol 1995;38:51-57.
12. Mahmoud H, Rivera G, Hancock M, et al. Low leukocyte counts with blast cells in cerebrospinal fluid of children with newly diagnosed acute lymphoblastic leukemia. New Engl J Med 1993; 329:314-319.
13. Lauer S, Shuster J, Kirchner P, et al. Prognostic significance of cerebrospinal fluid (CSF) lymphoblasts (LB) at diagnosis (dx) in children with acute lymphoblastic leukemia (ALL). Proc Am Soc Clin Oncol 1994;13:317.
14. Gilchrist G, Tubergen D, Sather H, et al. Low numbers of CSF blasts at diagnosis do not predict for the development of CNS leukemia in children with intermediate-risk acute lymphoblastic leukemia: A Children's Cancer Group Report. J Clin Oncol 1994; 12:2594-2600.
15. Heideman R, Packer R, Albright L, Freeman C, Rorke L. *Tumors of the central nervous system*. Philadelphia: Lippincott-Raven; 1997.
16. DeAngelis L. Current diagnosis and treatment of leptomeningeal metastasis. J Neurooncol 1998; 38:245-252.
17. Gajjar A, Fouladi M, Walter AW, et al. Comparison of lumbar and shunt cerebrospinal fluid specimens for cytologic detection of leptomeningeal disease in pediatric patients with brain tumors. J Clin Oncol 1999; 17:1825-1828.
18. Kallmes D, Gray L, Glass J. High-dose gadolinium-enhanced MRI for diagnosis of meningeal metastases. Neuroradiology 1998; 40:23-26.
19. Chamberlain M. Radioisotope CSF flow studies in leptomeningeal metastases. J Neurooncol 1998; 38:135-140.
20. Glantz M, Hall W, Cole B, et al. Diagnosis, management and survival of patients with leptomeningeal cancer based on cerebrospinal fluid-flow status. Cancer 1995; 75:2919-2931.

21. Bleyer W, Coccia P, Sather H, Level C, Lukens J, Niebrye D, Siegel S. Reduction in central nervous system leukemia with a pharmacokinetically derived intrathecal meth0trexate dosage regimen. J Clin Oncol 1983; 1:317-325.
22. Ritchey A, Pollock B, Lauer S, et al. Improved survival of children with isolated CNS relapse of acute lymphoblastic leukemia. J Clin Oncol 2000; 18:703.
23. Ritchey A, Pollock B, Lauer S, et al. Improved survival of children with isolated CNS relapse of acute lymphoblastic leukemia. J Clin Oncol 1999; 17:3745-3752.
24. Moser A, Adamson PC, Gillespie A, Poplack D, Balis F. Intraventricular concentration times time (C x T) methotrexate and cytarabine for patients with recurrent meningeal leukemia and lymphoma. Cancer 1999; 85:511-516.
25. Howell S, Gantz M, LaFollette S, Jaeckle K, Shapiro W. A controlled trial of Depocyt for the treatment of lymphomatous meningitis. In: Proc Am Soc Clin Oncol 1999:10a.
26. Kim S, Chatelut E, et al. Extended CSF cytarabine exposure following intrathecal administration of DTC 101. J Clin Oncol 1993; 11:2186-2193.
27. Blaney S, Poplack D. Neoplastic meningitis: diagnosis and treatment considerations. Medical Oncology 2000; 17:151-162.
28. van Besien K, Przepiorka D, Mehra R, et al. Impact of preexisting CNS involvement on the outcome of bone marrow transplantation in adult hematologic malignancies. J Clin Oncol 1996 14:3036-3042.
29. Shad A, Magrath I. Malignant non-Hodgkin's lymphomas in children. In: Pizzo P, Poplack D, eds. *Principles and Practice of Pediatric Oncology*. Philadelphia: Lippincott-raven; 1997.
30. Chamberlain M. A review of leptomeningeal metastases in pediatrics. J Child Neurol 1995; 10:191-199.
31. Grossman S, Moynihan T. Neurologic complications of systemic cancer; neoplastic meningitis. Neurol Clin 1991; 9:843-856.
32. Stanley P, Senac MJ, Segall H. Intraspinal seeding from intracranial tumors in children. Am J Neuroradiol 1984; 5:805-809.
33. Kandt R, Shinnar S, D'Souza B, et al. Cerebrospinal metastases in malignant childhood astrocytomas. J Neurooncol 1984; 2:123-128.
34. Civitello L, Packer R, Rorke L. Leptomeningeal dissemination of low-grade gliomas in childhood. Neurology 1988; 38:562-566.
35. Grabb P, Albright A, Pang D. Dissemination of supratentorial malignant gliomas via the cerebrospinal fluid in children. Neurosurgery. 1992; 30:64-71.
36. Wallner K, Wara W, Sheline G, Davis R. Intracranial ependymomas: Results of treatment with partial or whole brain irradiation without spinal irradiation. Int J Radiat Oncol Biol Phys 1983; 12:1937-1941.
37. Linstadt D, Wara W, Edwards M, Hudgins R, Sheline G. Radiotherapy of primary intracranial germinomas: The case against routine craniospinal irradiation. Int J Radiat Oncol Biol Phys 1988; 15:291-297.
38. Packer R, Siegel K, Sutton L, et al. Leptomeningeal dissemination of primary central nervous system tumors of childhood. Ann Neurol 1985; 18:217-221.
39. Allen J, Epstein F. Medulloblastoma and other primary malignant neuroectodermal tumors of the CNS. The effect of patients' age and extent of disease on prognosis. J Neurosurg 1982; 57:446-451.
40. Deutsch M, Reigel D. The value of myelography in the management of childhood medulloblastoma. Cancer 1980; 45:2194-2197.
41. Grill J, Renaux VK, Bulteau C, et al. Long-term intellectual outcome in children with posterior fossa tumors according to radiation doses and volumes. Int J Radiat Oncol Biol Phys 1999; 45:137-145.

42. Gajjar A, Kuhl J, Epelman S, Bailey C, Allen J. Chemotherapy of medulloblastoma. Childs Nerv Syst 1999; 15:554-562.
43. Packer RJ, Finlay JL. Chemotherapy for childhood medulloblastoma and primitive neuroectodermal tumors. Oncologist 1996; 1:381-393.
44. Zeltzer PM, Boyett JM, Finlay JL, et al. Metastasis stage, adjuvant treatment, and residual tumor are prognostic factors for medulloblastoma in children: conclusions from the Children's Cancer Group 921 randomized phase III study. J Clin Oncol 1999; 17:832-845.
45. Chamberlain M, Kormanik P. Chronic oral VP-16 for recurrent medulloblastoma. Pediatr Neuro 1997; 17:230-234.
46. Ashley D, Meier L, Kerby T, et al. Response of recurrent medulloblastoma to low-dose oral etoposide. J Clin Oncol 1996; 14:1922-1927.
47. Heideman RL. Overview of the treatment of infant central nervous system tumors: medulloblastoma as a model. J Pediatr Hematol Oncol 2001; 23:268-271.
48. Duffner P, Horowitz M, Krischer J. Postoperative chemotherapy and delayed radiation in children less than three years of age with malignant brain tumors. New Engl J Med 1993; 24:1725-1731.
49. Geyer J, Zeltzer PM, Boyett JM, et al. Survival of infants with primitive neuroectodermal tumors or malignant ependymomas of the CNS treated with eight drugs in 1 day: A report from the Children's Cancer Group. J Clin Oncol 1994; 12:1607-1615.
50. Mason W, Grovas A, Halpern S. Intensive chemotherapy and bone marrow rescue for young children with newly diagnosed malignant brain tumors. J Clin Oncol 1998; 16:210-221.
51. Walter AW, Mulhern RK, Gajjar A. Survival and neurodevelopmental outcome of young children with medulloblastoma at St. Jude Children's Research Hospital. J Clin Oncol 1999;17:3720-3728.
52. Pollack I, Gerszten P, Martinez A, et al. Intracranial ependymomas of childhood: long-term outcome and prognostic factors. Neurosurgery 1995;37: 655-667.
53. Packer R, Allen J, Nielsen S, Petito C, Deck M, Jereb B. Brainstem glioma: clinical manifestations of meningeal gliomatosis. *Ann Neurol* 1983;14:177-182.
54. Pollack I, Hurtt M, Pang D, Albright A. Dissemination of low grade intracranial astrocytomas in children. Cancer 1994;73:2869-2878.
55. Dirks P, Jay V, Becker L, Drake J, Humphrey R, Hoffman H, Ruthka J. Development of anaplastic changes in low-grade astrocytomas of childhood. *Neurosurgery* 1994;34:68-78.
56. Obana W, Cogen P, Davis R, Edwards M. Metastatic juvenile pilocytic astrocytoma. Case report. J Neurosurg 1991;75:972-975.
57. Bruggers C, Friedman H, Phillips P, et al. Leptomeningeal dissemination of optic pathway gliomas in three children. Am J Ophthalmol 1991; 111:719-723.
58. Tamura M, Zama A, Kurihara H, et al. Management of recurrent pilocytic astrocytoma with leptomeningeal dissemination of childhood. Child's Nerv Syst 1998; 14:617-622.
59. Shapiro K, Shulman K. Spinal cord seeding from cerebellar astrocytomas. Child's Brain 1976; 2:177-186.
60. Kocks W, Kalff R, Reinhardt V, Grote W, Hilke J. Spinal metastasis of pilocytic astrocytoma of the chiasma opticum. *Child's Nerv Syst* 1989; 5:118-120.
61. Paulino A, Thomas C, Slomiany D, Suarez C. Diffuse malignant leptomeningeal gliomatosis in a child: A case report and review of the literature. Am J Clin Oncol 1999; 22:243-246.
62. Dietrich P-Y, Aapro M, Rieder A, Pizzolato G. Primary diffuse leptomeningeal gliomatosis (PDLG): a neoplastic cause of chronic meningitis. J Neurooncol 1993; 15:275-283.
63. Ho K, Hoschner J, Wolfe D. Primary leptomeningeal gliomatosis. Symptoms suggestive of meningitis. Arch Neurol 1981; 38:662-666.
64. Ng H-K, Poon W-S. Diffuse leptomeningeal gliomatosis with oligodendroglioma. Pathology 1999; 31:59-63.

65. Kitahara M, Katakura R, Wada T, Maniki T, Suzuki J. Diffuse form of primary leptomeningeal gliomatosis. J Neurosurg 1985; 63:283-287.
66. Jennings M, Gelman R, Hochberg F. Intracranial germ-cell tumors: Natural history and pathogenesis. J Neurosurg 1985; 63:155-167.
67. Buckner J, Peethambaram P, Smithson W, et al. Phase II trial of primary chemotherapy followed by reduced-dose radiation for CNS germ cell tumors. J Clin Oncol 1999; 17:933-940.
68. Allen J, Kim J, Packer R. Neoadjuvant chemotherapy for newly diagnosed germ-cell tumors of the central nervous system. J Neurosurg 1987; 67:65-70.
69. Chow E, Reardon D, Shah A, et al T. Pediatric choroid plexus neoplasms. Int J Radiation Oncology Biol Phys 1999; 44:249-254.
70. Allen J, Wisoff J, Helson L, Pearce J, Arenson E. Choroid plexus carcinoma-- responses to chemotherapy alone in newly diagnosed young children. J Neurooncol 1992; 12:69-74.
71. Boyd M, Steinbok P. Choroid plexus tumors: Problems in diagnosis and management. J Neurosurg 1987; 66:800-805.
72. Sheikh B, Siqueira E, Dayel F. Meningioma in children: A report of nine cases and review of the literature. Surg Neurol 1996; 45:328-335.
73. Chan R, Thompson G. Intracranial meningiomas in childhood. Surg Neurol 1984; 21:319-322.
74. Crouse S, Berg B. Intracranial meningiomas in childhood and adolescence. Neurology 1972; 22:135-141.
75. Diaz P, Maillo A, Morales F, Gomez-Moreta J, Hernandez J. Multiple meningiomas of the fourth ventricle in infancy: case report. Neurosurgery 1990;26: 1057-1060.
76. Donovan W, Govoni A. An 11 year-old boy with a history of AML and new onset headaches. Clinical Imaging 1992; 16:272-276.
77. Hope J, Armstrong D, Babyn P, et al. Primary meningeal tumors in children: correlation of clinical and CT findings with histologic type and prognosis. Am J Neuroradiol 1992; 13:1353-1364.
78. Kamiya K, Inagawa T, Nagasako R. Malignant intraventricular meningioma with spinal metastasis through the cerebrospinal fluid. Surg Neurol 1989; 32:213-218.
79. Miller A, Ramsden F. Malignant meningioma with extracranial metastases and seeding of the subarachnoid space and the ventricles. Pathol Eur 1972; 7:167-175.
80. Jallo G, Kothbauer K, Silvera V, Epstein F. Intraspinal clear cell meningioma: Diagnosis and management: Report of two cases. Neurosurgery 2001; 48:218-222.
81. Lee W, Chang K-H, Cho G, et al. MR Imaging features of clear-cell meningioma with diffuse leptomeningeal seeding. Am J Neuroradiol 2000; 21:130-132.
82. Meli F, Boccaleri C, Manzitti J, Lylyk P. Meningeal dissemination of retinoblastoma: CT findings in eight patients. AJNR. 1990;11:983-986.
83. Blatt J, Fitz C, Mirro, Jr J. Recognition of central nervous system metastases in children with metastatic primary extracranial neuroblastoma. Pediatr Hematol Oncol 1997; 14:233-241.
84. Kellie S, Hayes F, Bowman L, et al. Primary extracranial neuroblastoma with central nervous system metastases characterization by clinicopathologic findings and neuroimaging. Cancer 1991; 68:1999-2006.
85. Rohrlich P, Hartmann O, Couanet D, et al. Localizations neuro-meningees metastatiques secondaires dans les neuroblastomes de l'enfant. Arch Fr Pediatr 1989; 46:5-10.
86. Shaw P, Eden T. Neuroblastoma with intracranial involvement: an ENSG study. Med Pediatr Oncol 1992; 20:149-155.
87. Parasuraman S, Langston J, Rao B, et al. Brain metastases in pediatric Ewing's sarcoma and rhabdomyosarcoma: The St. Jude Children's Research Hospital experience. J Pediatr Hematol Oncol 1999; 21:370-377.

88. Allcutt D, Michowicz M, Weitzman S, et al. Primary leptomeningeal melanoma: an unusually aggressive tumor in childhood. Neurosurg 1993; 32:721-729.
89. Rodriguez-Galindo C, Pappo A, Kaste S, et al. Brain metastases in children with melanoma. Cancer 1997; 79:2440-2445.
90. Trigg M, Makuch R, Glaubiger D. Actuarial risk of isolated CNS involvement in Ewing's sarcoma following prophylactic cranial irradiation and intrathecal methotrexate. Int J Radiation Oncology Biol Phys 1985; 11:699-702.
91. Yu L, Craver R, Baliga M, et al. Isolated CNS involvement in Ewing's sarcoma. Med Pediatr Oncol 1990; 18:354-358.
92. Wharam MJ. Rhabdomyosarcoma of parameningeal sites. Semin Radiat Oncol 1997; 7:212-216.
93. Russell D, Rubinstein L. *Pathology of Tumours of the Nervous System*. 3d ed. Baltimore: Williams & Wilkins; 1971.
94. Krill A. *Krill's Hereditary Retinal and Choroidal Diseases*. New York: Harper & Row; 1977.
95. Davis P, Friedman N, Fry S, Malko J, Hoffman JJ, Braun I. Leptomeningeal metastasis: MR imaging. Radiology 1987; 163:449-454.
96. Donaldson S, Egbert E, Lee W-H. Retinoblastoma. In: Pizzo P, Poplack P, eds. *Principles and Practice of Pediatric Oncology*. Philadelphia: J.B. Lippincott Co; 1989:683-696.
97. Kramer K, Kushner B, Heller G, Cheung N-K. Neuroblastoma metastatic to the central nervous system. Cancer 2001; 91:1510-1519.
98. Trigg M, Glaubiger D, Nesbit M. The frequency of isolated CNS involvement in Ewing's sarcoma. Cancer 1982; 49:2404-2409.
99. Makin G, Eden O, Lashford L, et al. Leptomeningeal melanoma in childhood. Cancer 1999; 86:878-886.
100. Poe L, Roitberg D, Galyon D. Neurocutaneous melanosis presenting as an intradural mass of the cervical canal: magnetic resonance features and the presence of melanin as a clue to diagnosis: case report. Neurosurgery 1994; 35:741-743.
101. Eaves F, Burstein F, Hudgins R, Cohen S, Papciack M. Primary temporal melanoma without diffuse leptomeningeal involvement: variant of neurocutaneous melanosis. Plastic Reconstr Surg. 1995;95:133-136.
102. Frieden I, Williams M, Barkovich A. Giant congenital melanocytic nevi: brain magnetic resonance findings in neurologically asymptomatic children. J Am Acad Dermatol 1994; 31:423-429.
103. Blasberg R, Patlak C, Fenstermacher J. Intrathecal chemotherapy brain tissue profiles after ventriculo-cisternal perfusion. Pharm Exp Ther 1975; 195:73-83.
104. Poplack D, Bleyer W, Horowitz M. *Pharmacology of antineoplastic agents in cerebrospinal fluid*. New York: Plenum Press; 1980.
105. Kaplan R, Wiernik P. Neurotoxicity of antineoplastic drugs. Semin Oncol 1982; 9:103-130.
106. Blaney S, Poplack D. Pharmacologic strategies for the treatment of meningeal malignancy. Investigational New Drugs 1996; 14:69-85.
107. Voorhess M, Brecker M, Glickman A, et al. Hypothalamic-pituitary function of children with acute lymphocytic leukemia after three forms of central nervous system prophylaxis. A retrospective study. Cancer 1986; 57:1287-1291.
108. Pasqualini T, McCalla J, Berg S, et al. Subtle primary hypothyroidism in patients treated for acute lymphoblastic leukemia. Acta Endocrinol *(Copenh)* 1991; 124:375-380.
109. Blatt J, Bercu B, Gillin J, Mendelson W, Poplack D. Reduced pulsatile growth hormone secretion in children after therapy for acute lympoblastic leukemia. J Pediatr 1984; 104:182-186.

110. Moss H, Nannis E, Poplack D. The effects of prophylactic treatment of the central nervous system on the intellectual functioning of children with acute lymphocytic leukemia. Am J Med 1981; 71:47-52.
111. Paolucci G, Rosito P. *Adverse sequelae of central nervous system prophylaxis in acute lymphoblastic leukemia*. Boston: Martinus Nijhoff; 1983.
112. Poplack D. *Evaluation of adverse sequelae of central nervous sustem prophylaxis in acute lymphoblstic leukemia*. Boston: Martinus Nijhoff; 1983.
113. Radcliff J, Packer R, Atkins T, et al. Prospective study of cognitive function in children with medulloblastoma receiving whole brain radiotherapy and chemotherapy. Ann Neurol 1992; 32:551-555.
114. Johnson D, McGabe M, Nicholson H, et al. Quality of long-term survival in young children with medulloblastoma. J Neurosurg 1994; 80:1004-1010.
115. MacLean W, Noll R, Stehbens J, et al. Neuropsychological effects of cranial irradiation in young children with acute lymphoblastic leukemia 9 months after diagnosis. Arch Neurol 1995; 52:156-160.

Chapter 7

NEUROSURGICAL INTERVENTIONS FOR LEPTOMENINGEAL TUMOR

Jeffrey P. Greenfield[1,2] and Mark H. Bilsky[1,2]
[1]*Department of Surgery, Neurosurgery Service, Memorial Sloan-Kettering Cancer Center, 1275 York Avenue, New York, NY 10021*; [2]*Department of Neurological Surgery, New York Presbyterian Hospital, 525 E. 68th Street, New York, NY 10021.*

Abstract: Nonsurgical modalities remain the keystone to treatment and control of leptomeningeal tumor. However, neurosurgical consultation is often required for placement of Ommaya reservoirs and ventriculoperitoneal shunts. In this chapter, the utility of these devices, as well as their common complications will be presented. The aim will be to familiarize non-surgical providers with the indications for and complications associated with these neurosurgical procedures as a component of the adjuvant treatment of leptomeningeal disease.

Keywords: Intraventricular chemotherapy; Ommaya reservoir; ventriculo-peritoneal shunt; leptomeningeal disease; hydrocephalus.

1. INTRODUCTION

Chemotherapy and radiation are the standard treatments for leptomeningeal disease. Intrathecal (IT) chemotherapy alone, or in combination with systemic chemotherapy[1] including methotrexate, cytarabine[2] (Ara-C), and thiotepa[3], are used to treat patients with lymphoma, leukemia, and metastatic solid tumors, such as breast carcinoma. More recently, IT, targeted radioimmunotherapy, such as ^{131}I-3F8[4], has been explored for leptomeningeal tumors that are GD2-positive.

Leptomeningeal disease, by definition, is disseminated along the spinal axis and is not resectable (Fig.1).

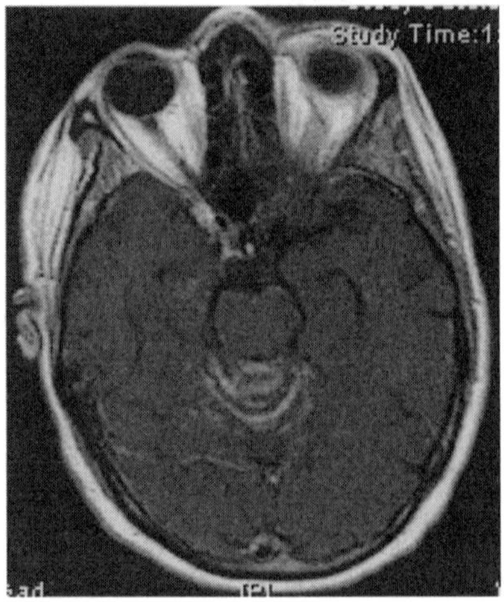

Figure 1. Leptomeningeal Disease: Contrast-enhanced T1 MRI (A,B), axial images demonstrating leptomeningeal enhancement in a patient who underwent Ommaya reservoir placement for intrathecal chemotherapy.

Due to the lack of discreet, bulky tumor, neurosurgeons have a limited role in treating this disseminated disease. Their involvement usually is requested when oncologists are considering the placement of a ventricular access device. These devices are designed to enhance IT drug delivery and to more efficiently and precisely monitor treatment efficacy. Access to the cerebrospinal fluid (CSF) for delivery of chemotherapy can be achieved either by performing repeated spinal taps, or by placement of a permanent catheter into the intraventricular space. These catheters are connected to low-profile, subcutaneous reservoirs which may be easily accessed transcutaneously with small bore needles (Fig. 2).

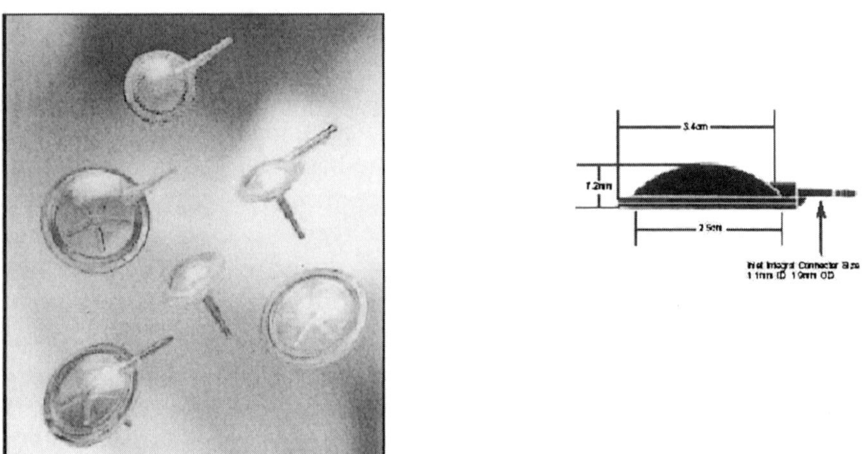

Figure 2. Ommaya reservoir: Low-profile subcutaneous reservoir connected to intraventricular catheters allow easy access to CSF for intermittent chemotherapy infusions. *Figure 2 images courtesy of Integra LifeSciences Corporation*

The first such reservoir was utilized in 1963 and has since borne the name of its innovator, Dr. A.K. Ommaya.[5] Ommaya reservoirs have several advantages over repeated spinal taps. For the patient, an obvious advantage is the increased convenience and comfort of accessing an Ommaya reservoir when compared with repeated lumbar spinal taps. For the oncologist, whose goal is effective drug delivery, intraventricular delivery of chemotherapy has a better volume of distribution than lumbar puncture. A further advantage is the ease with which hydrocephalus, a condition that develops in approximately 10% of patients with leptomeningeal disease, can be managed once an Ommaya reservoir has been placed[6].

1.1 Techniques for catheter placement

The precise placement of intraventricular catheters is of paramount importance when considering the surgical nuances of implanting Ommaya reservoirs. Proper catheter placement is important to avoid damaging eloquent cortex or subcortical structures along the catheter's trajectory. In addition, proper targeting of the catheter so that its tip is within the ventricle is crucial to avoid administering toxic chemotherapy directly into brain parenchyma. Inadvertent administration of chemotherapy into brain parenchyma can cause mild to severe leukoencephalopathy, the destruction of the myelin sheaths which cover nerve fibers. Ideally, the ventricular catheter is placed so that all of the catheter outlet holes, typically extending two centimeters from the catheter tip, are within the ventricular compartment. This goal is readily achieved by placing the catheter tip at the ipsilateral foramen of Monro. In addition to ensuring that all of the outlet holes are within the CSF space, catheter tip placement at the foramen of Monro also lessens the likelihood of the catheter tip becoming entangled in the choroid plexus or septal veins causing hemorrhage at initial surgery or revision. Intraoperative confirmation of the catheter tip position can be achieved using a variety of techniques, including pneumoencephalography, frame-based or frameless stereotaxy[7], and/or endoscopy.[6,8] Postoperative CT confirmation is routinely obtained prior to chemotherapy delivery. If safe delivery of chemotherapy remains a concern due to equivocal CT confirmation, radioactive tracer studies can be performed, followed by whole brain scintography at various time-points (up to 24 hours) to document safe tracer distribution throughout the CSF, but excluding brain parenchyma.

The surgical technique for Ommaya reservoir placement utilizing either pneumoencephalography or frameless stereotaxy will be briefly described. For either method, a horseshoe shaped incision is centered 10 cms from the nasion and 3 cms from the midline (mid-pupillary line) on the right (non-dominant) side. A burr hole is created using a craniotome. A subgaleal pocket is created using blunt dissection posterior to the incision and the Ommaya reservoir is inserted. The dura is coagulated using bipolar cautery and opened with an 11 blade.

When using pneumoencephalography, the ventricular catheter is initially placed using the Ghajar guide (Neurodynamics, New York, NY) or free–hand based on anatomic landmarks. The catheter tip is typically placed 5.5 cms from the inner table of the skull. Approximately 10 mls of CSF are drained and sent for cytology. Air is then injected into the catheter under continuous fluoroscopy until both the ipsilateral lateral ventricle and third ventricle are air-filled (Fig. 3A, 3B).

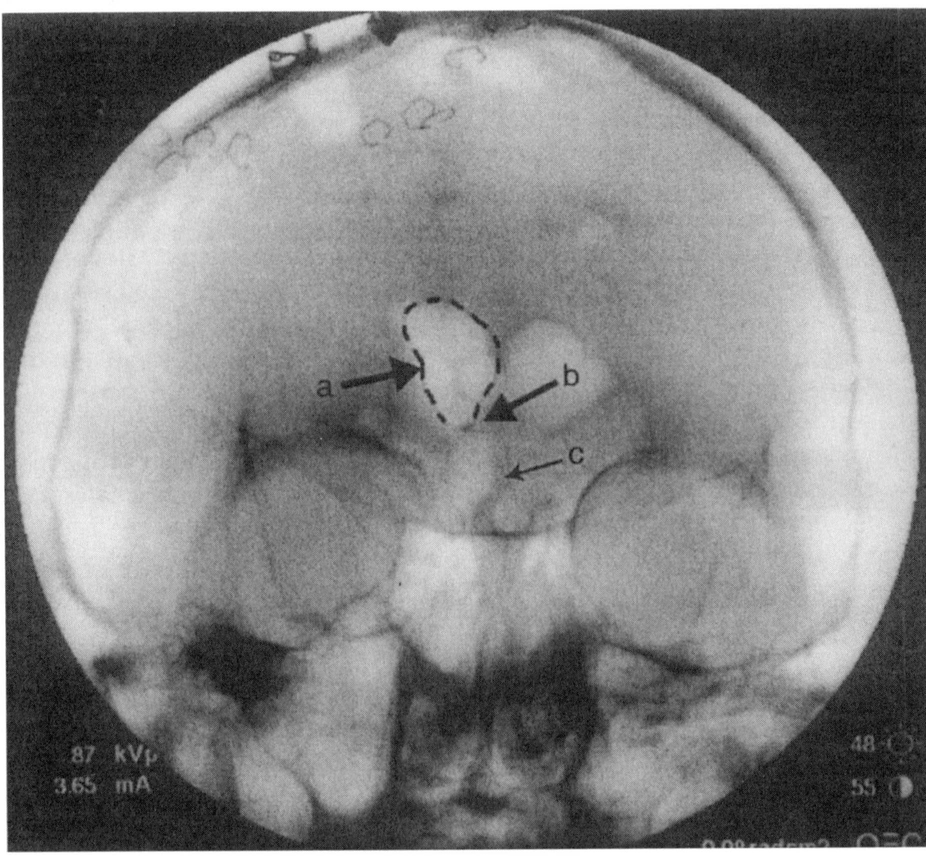

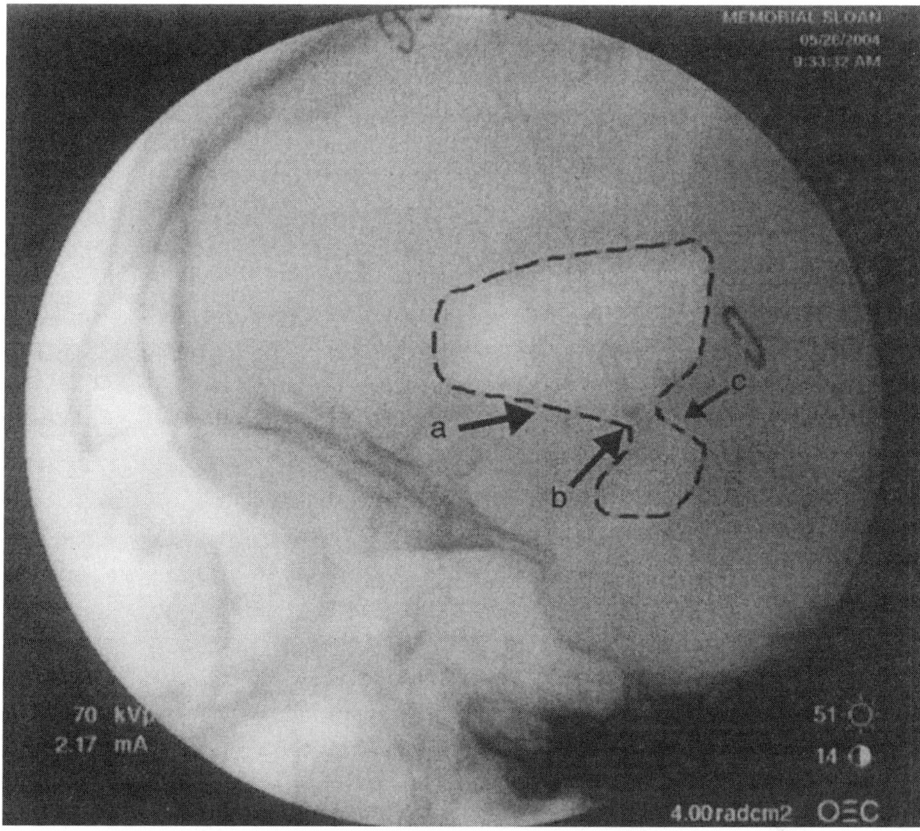

Figure 3. Fluoroscopic Ommaya placement: Intraoperative A/P (A: top panel), and lateral (B: bottom panel), fluoroscopic images demonstrating air-filled right lateral ventricle (a). The catheter tip (b) can be seen approaching the Foramen of Monroe (c).

A vascular clip is placed at the proximal end of the ventricular catheter, and the catheter is manually manipulated until the tip is placed at the ipsilateral foramen of Monro, typically 5.8 cms from the inner table of the skull. Catheter lengths greater than 6 cms usually suggest improper catheter positioning often in the contralateral caudate nucleus, basilar cisterns, or even contralateral Sylvian fissure. Fluoroscopy can help redirect the catheter into the proper trajectory in real time. Having placed the catheter at the desired target, the catheter is cut and secured to a right angle connector on the Ommaya reservoir with a 2-0 silk tie. The right angle connector is then secured to the skull through a drill hole in the posterior aspect of the burr hole with a 2-0 silk stitch. The wound is irrigated with antibiotic solution and closed in two layers.

For frameless stereotaxy, i.e., without intraoperative fluoroscopy, patients undergo pre-operative CT scans with fiducial markers. Once in the operating room, they are placed into a rigid frame using skull pins, followed by registration to the stereotactic system. The opening of the skull and dura is identical to the prior technique. However, the placement of the catheter is then directed using the ventricular catheter probe to the indicated depth by aligning the trajectory in two planes using the trajectory mode and guidance views on the stereotactic system (Fig. 4). Once positioned correctly, the catheter and reservoir are secured as described above. Either method should ensure catheter placement at the foramen of Monro. Our preferred method remains intraoperative pneumoencephalography, which allows one to achieve a real time intraoperative image that also demonstrates patency of the ventricular catheter.

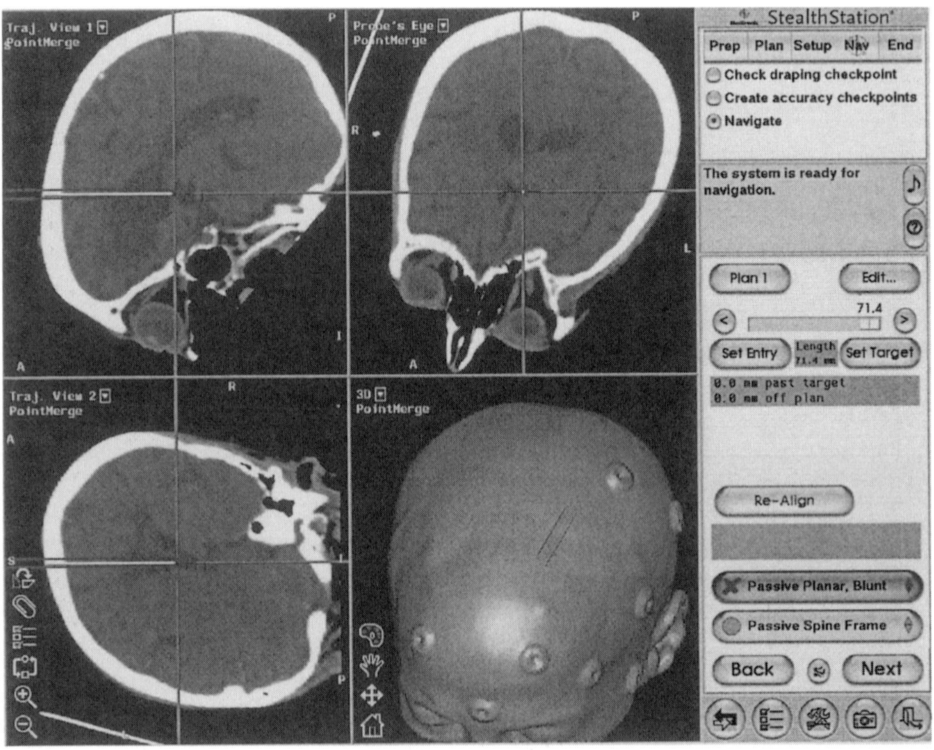

Figure 4. Frameless Stereotaxy for Ommaya Placement: Intraoperative Stealth Station screen demonstrating real-time three-dimensional view of the catheter trajectory necessary to place the tip at the Foramen of Monroe

1.2 Hydrocephalus

At Memorial Sloan-Kettering Cancer Center (MSKCC), approximately 10% of patients referred for placement of Ommaya reservoirs have or develop hydrocephalus.[6] This is typically communicating hydrocephalus, resulting from occlusion of the arachnoid granulations necessary for CSF resorption into the venous system or from basilar carcinomatous meningitis. On rare occasions patients will develop a non-communicating hydrocephalus secondary to an obstructing lesion at the foramen of Monro, Sylvian aqueduct, or fourth ventricle. When obstruction occurs of either communicating or non-communicating variants, the ventricles will normally dilate making the diagnosis evident. However, a small percentage of patients will have non-compliant, small or "slit" ventricles which result in markedly elevated intracranial pressure without radiographically-apparent hydrocephalus. Patients with elevated intracranial pressure often present with severe headaches, emesis, and altered levels of consciousness in addition to focal neurologic deficits.

Acute hydrocephalus in patients with leptomeningeal disease is an urgent situation requiring a ventriculoperitoneal shunt (Fig. 5).

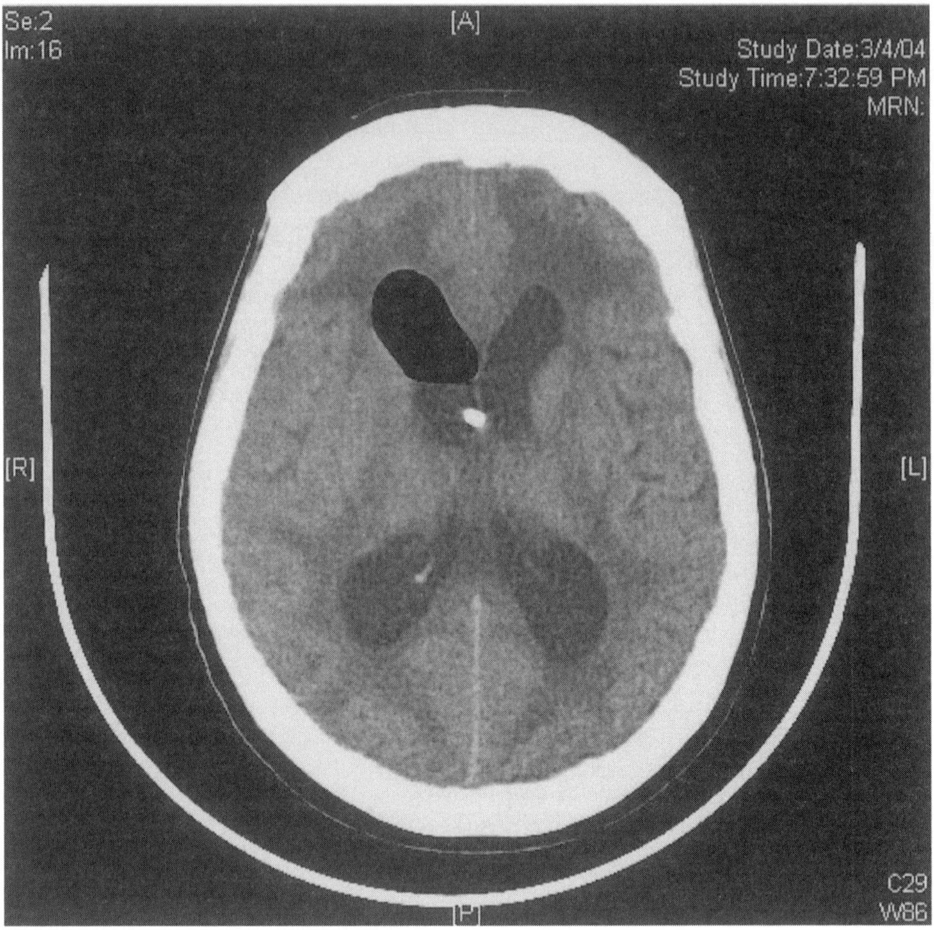

Figure 5. Hydrocephalus and Leptomeningeal Disease: Non-contrast CT showing ventricular dilation in a patient undergoing Ommaya reservoir placement for leptomeningeal disease.

Patients who develop hydrocephalus and already have had an Ommaya reservoir placed have the advantage of being able to have a neurosurgeon connect a shunt valve and peritoneal catheter sequentially to their reservoir, thereby avoiding a second intracranial surgery. Conversely, for patients with hydrocephalus who later require IT chemotherapy for treatment of leptomeningeal disease, the option of turning up a programmable valve on a ventriculoperitoneal shunt to allow CSF drug delivery and then turning the valve back to the original setting to permit CSF drainage is invaluable. On-off valves were used for many to years to achieve this purpose, but they were relatively cumbersome to use and unreliable. Over the past five years at MSKCC, we have utilized the Codman-Hakim programmable valve (Johnson and Johnson, Raynham, MA), which uses a magnet to control the resistance in the valve (Fig. 6).

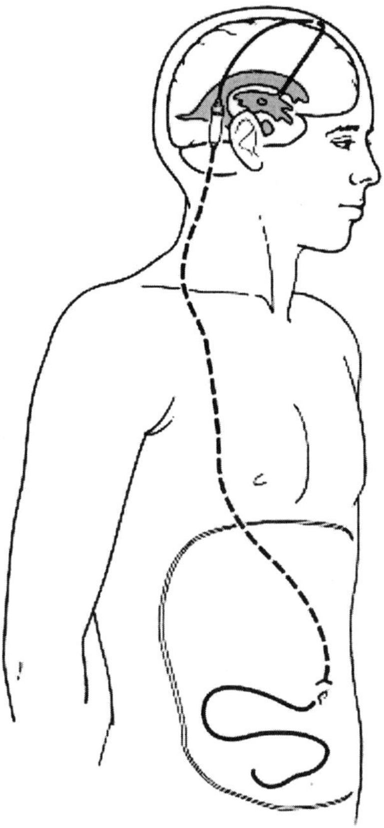

Figure 6. Conversion of an Ommaya Reservoir to Ventriculoperitoneal Shunt: Placement of Ommaya catheter with convertible reservoir (A), allows easy conversion to a Ventriculoperitoneal shunt (B), while still allowing intermittent chemotherapy infusions.
Figure 6b image courtesy of Integra Life Sciences Corporation

During drug delivery, the valve is placed to the highest setting and then reset after four hours. A plain radiograph of the skull will show that the valve has been reset. The valve can be reset repeatedly without damaging the mechanism. One patient has been treated for leptomeningeal disease from metastatic breast carcinoma every other week for two years without encountering any difficulties with the valve.

Of practical note for oncologists and neurologists, it should be emphasized that when instilling chemotherapy, it is necessary to withdraw CSF equal to the amount to be instilled. Difficulty in obtaining CSF can be secondary to slit or small ventricles. This difficulty can be remedied by placing the patient in Trendelenburg position and waiting for CSF to accumulate. It is also worth mentioning endoscopic third ventriculostomies. Their recent increase in popularity has made it more likely that well-informed patients will inquire about the possibility of having the procedure done in lieu of one requiring permanent hardware. While third ventriculostomy has gained acceptance for the treatment of many types of hydrocephalus, it is not an option in patients with leptomeningeal tumor both because it is ineffective in treating communicating hydrocephalus and does not address the need for a chemotherapy delivery system.

2. COMPLICATIONS

Risks of Ommaya catheter placement include hemorrhage, poor positioning and the sequelae of intraparenchymal chemotherapy toxicity, malfunction and infection.[9] The rate of intraventricular hemorrhage in published series is between 1 to 2.8%.[2,4,5,6] Hemorrhages in the cancer population may be related to hematologic abnormalities, such as thrombocytopenia or disseminated intravascular coagulopathy related to the primary cancer or treatment related effects. These risks may be long-standing and occur up to a month after placement, making the coordination of chemotherapy regimens and their expected platelet or white blood cell count nadirs to avoid surgery of utmost importance. For minor abnormalities that are correctable, such as thrombocytopenia, the persistent need for transfusion to keep platelets elevated is a relative contraindication as is need for full anticoagulation.

Despite repeated reservoir punctures for chemotherapy delivery, the development of bacterial meningitis is relatively uncommon after Ommaya placement. Quoted infection rates vary between 1.9 to 9% typically secondary to gram-positive organisms.[6,10,11,12,13,14] The most common organism is *Staphylococcus epidermidis*. Most infections can be treated without removing the catheter using a combination of systemic and intrathecal antibiotics, however, persistently positive cultures necessitate hardware removal. Wound dehiscence with exposed hardware most commonly occurs when the Ommaya reservoir is positioned within the incision. Our preference is to use an Ommaya with a right angle connector that allows the reservoir to be positioned posterior to the incision. After placement of over 200 catheters, we have not had any complications involving hardware exposure.

Intraventricular administration of chemotherapy from poorly positioned catheters may result in chemical meningitis in up to 50% of patients undergoing therapy, regardless of the drug administered. Chemical meningitis is heralded by low-grade fever, headache, nausea, vomiting, meningismus and photophobia. CSF cytology typically shows a sterile pleocytosis. Symptoms are often short-lived with the administration of low-dose oral steroids.

Leukoencephalopathy secondary to chemotherapy can occur months to years after the administration of the intraventricular drug.[15] Symptoms cover the spectrum of neurologic findings, from the subtle: mental status changes, field deficits and peripheral neuropathies, to the extreme: focal seizures and progression to coma and death. Neuropathologic findings of leukoencephalopathy are similarly diverse in their severity and distribution although in most, the white matter is affected by severe myelin pallor, edema and prominent macrophage infiltrates. Radiographically, mild chemotherapy-induced leukoencephalopathy shows no contrast enhancement, but rather mild-to-moderate diffuse high signal in deep white matter which usually resolves. In more severe cases, initial T2-weighted images may show discreet areas of high signal which may spread and coalesce to involve the entire white matter. Small irregular low-signal foci on T2-weighted images can be seen within the high-signal lesions.[16]

3. CONCLUSIONS

The treatment of leptomeningeal tumor by multiple modalities is evolving. Neurosurgical intervention is usually limited to placement of ventricular access devices or ventricular shunts. Placement of Ommaya reservoirs is often an integral part of providing effective concentrations of chemotherapeutics to otherwise unresectable metastatic disease within the central nervous system. While precise reservoir placement has become very reliable using modern navigational techniques, limiting the most serious side effects of leukoencephalopathy, other side effects such as hemorrhage and infection especially in the myelosuppressed and immunosuppressed patient populations, must be seriously weighted against the benefits of beginning IT chemotherapy.

REFERENCES

1. Pels H, Schmidt-Wolf IG, Glasmacher A, et al. Primary central nervous system lymphoma: results of a pilot and phase II study of systemic and intraventricular chemotherapy with deferred radiotherapy. J Clin Oncol 2003; 21:4489-95.
2. Esteva FJ, Soh, LT, Holmes FA, et al. Phase II trial and pharmacokinetic evaluation of cytosine arabinoside for leptomeningeal metastases from breast cancer. Cancer Chemother Pharmacol 2000; 46:382-6.
3. Witham TF, Fukui MB, Meltzer CC, et al. Survival of patients with high grade glioma treated with intrathecal thio triethylenephosphoramide for ependymal or leptomeningeal gliomatosis. Cancer 1999; 86:1347-53.
4. Kramer K, Cheung NK, Humm JL, et al. Targeted radioimmunotherapy for leptomeningeal cancer using (131)I-3F8. Med Pediatr Oncol 2000; 35:716-8.
5. Witorsch P, Williams TW Jr, Ommaya AK, Utz JP. Intraventricular administration of amphotericin B. Use of subcutaneous reservoir in four patients with mycotic meningitis. JAMA 1965; 194:699-702.
6. Sandberg DI, Bilsky MH, Souweidane MM, Bzdil J, Gutin PH. Ommaya reservoirs for the treatment of leptomeningeal metastases. Neurosurgery 2000; 47:49-54.
7. Greenfield JP, Schwartz TH. Frameless stereotaxy for Ommaya Reservoirs. Neurosurgery 2004 [*Submitted for publication*].
8. Al-Anazi A, Bernstein M. Modified stereotactic insertion of the Ommaya reservoir. Technical note. J Neurosurg 2000; 92:1050-2.
9. Cheshire WP, Ehle AL. Hemiparkinsonism as a complication of an Ommaya reservoir. Case report. J. Neurosurg 1990; 73:774-6.
10. Galicich JH, Guido LJ. Ommaya device in carcinomatous and leukemic meningitis: surgical experience in 45 cases. Surg Clin North Am 1974; 54:915-22.
11. Lishner M, Perrin RG, Feld R, et al. Complications associated with Ommaya reservoirs in patients with cancer. The Princess Margaret Hospital experience and a review of the literature.. Arch Intern Med 1990; 150:173-6.
12. Obbens EA, Leavens ME, Beal JW, Lee YY. Ommaya reservoirs in 387 cancer patients: a 15-year experience. Neurology 1985; 35:1274-8.
13. Mehta BM, Glass JP, Shapiro WR. Serum and cerebrospinal fluid distribution of 5-methyltetrahydrofolate after intravenous calcium leucovorin and intra-Ommaya methotrexate administration in patients with meningeal carcinomatosis. Cancer Res 1983; 43:435-8.
14. Shapiro WR, Young DF, Mehta MB. Methotrexate: distribution in cerebrospinal fluid after intravenous, ventricular and lumbar injections. N Engl J Med 1975; ;293:161-6.
15. Lemann W, Wiley RG, Posner JB. Leukoencephalopathy complicating intraventricular catheters: clinical, radiographic and pathologic study of 10 cases. J Neurooncol 1988; 6:67-74.
16. Oka M, Terae S, Kobayashi R, et al. MRI in methotrexate-related leukoencephalopathy: Disseminated necrotizing leukoencephalopathy in comparison with mild leukoencephalopathy. Neuroradiology 2003; 45:493-7.

FIGURE LEGENDS

Figure 1. Leptomeningeal Disease: Contrast-enhanced T1 MRI (A,B), axial images demonstrating leptomeningeal enhancement in a patient who underwent Ommaya reservoir placement for intrathecal chemotherapy.

Figure 2. Ommaya reservoir: Low-profile subcutaneous reservoir connected to intraventricular catheters allow easy access to CSF for intermittent chemotherapy infusions. *Figure 2 images courtesy of Integra LifeSciences Corporation*

Figure 3. Fluoroscopic Ommaya placement: Intraoperative A/P (A), and lateral (B), fluoroscopic images demonstrating air-filled right lateral ventricle (a). The catheter tip (b) can be seen approaching the Foramen of Monroe (c).

Figure 4. Frameless Stereotaxy for Ommaya Placement: Intraoperative Stealth Station screen demonstrating real-time three-dimensional view of the catheter trajectory necessary to place the tip at the Foramen of Monroe

Figure 5. Hydrocephalus and Leptomeningeal Disease: Non-contrast CT showing ventricular dilation in a patient undergoing Ommaya reservoir placement for leptomeningeal disease.

Figure 6. Conversion of an Ommaya Reservoir to Ventriculoperitoneal Shunt: Placement of Ommaya catheter with convertible reservoir (A), allows easy conversion to a Ventriculoperitoneal shunt (B), while still allowing intermittent chemotherapy infusions.
Figure 6b image courtesy of Integra Life Sciences Corporation

Chapter 8

CURRENT TREATMENT OF LEPTOMENINGEAL METASTASES: SYSTEMIC CHEMOTHERAPY, INTRATHECAL CHEMOTHERAPY AND SYMPTOM MANAGEMENT

Stacey L. Berg, M.D., Marc C. Chamberlain, M.D.
Norris Cancer Center, University of Southern California, Los Angeles, Ca. 90089

Abstract: Treatment of leptomeningeal metastases is multifaceted and includes symptomatic therapy, intrathecal and systemic chemotherapy, and radiotherapy. As the majority of patients have widespread incurable systemic tumor, treatment is predominantly palliative; however, some patients with leukemia, lymphoma or breast cancer may have prolonged remissions and the possibility of cure.

Keywords: Intrathecal chemotherapy; systemic chemotherapy; CSF flow; breast cancer; methotrexate, cytarabine; thiotepa.

1. INTRODUCTION

Many common cancers, including leukemia, carcinomas of the lung, breast, gastrointestinal tract, and brain tumors metastasize to the leptomeninges.[1-20] Because the cerebrospinal fluid (CSF) flows between the pia mater and the arachnoid in the subarachnoid space, tumor involving one part of the leptomeninges spreads easily throughout the neuraxis.[21,22] Thus, leptomeningeal metastasis is usually considered a diffuse disease of the central nervous system (CNS) even when measurable disease appears to be limited.

The diffuse nature of leptomeningeal carcinomatosis implies that therapy must be directed to the entire CNS if tumor control is the desired outcome.[23-27] Treatment of neoplastic meningitis is therefore multimodal and encompasses the entire neuraxis including the ventricular system, base of brain cisterns and the spinal subarachnoid space[1-19] (Table 1) (Table 2) (Fig. 1).

Table 1: Leptomeningeal Metastases: Treatment Modalities

Modality	**Comments**
Corticosteroids	Temporary symptom relief in patients with bulky intraparenchymal metastasis resulting in raised intracranial pressure
Radiotherapy	Bulky lesions (symptomatic and/or seen on imaging)
and sites of CSF	
Limited-field	flow obstruction
Craniospinal	
Chemotherapy	Treats entire neuraxis
Regional	Pharmacokinetic advantages
Antimetabolites	
Alkylating agents	
Systemic	Improved drug distribution
High dose IV: Methotrexate, cytarabine, thio-TEPA	
Surgery	
Ommaya reservoir	
CSF diversion	
Immunotherapy	Investigational
Regional	

Table-2: Standard therapy for leptomeningeal metastasis

- Radiotherapy to sites of symptomatic and bulky disease and to sites of CSF flow obstruction
- Intra-CSF chemotherapy (one of the following; may be used sequentially in patients failing prior therapy)
    - Methotrexate
    - Cytarabine
    - Thio-TEPA
- Concurrent systemic treatment of primary tumor

Figure 1: TREATMENT ALGORITHM OF NEOPLASTIC MENINGITIS

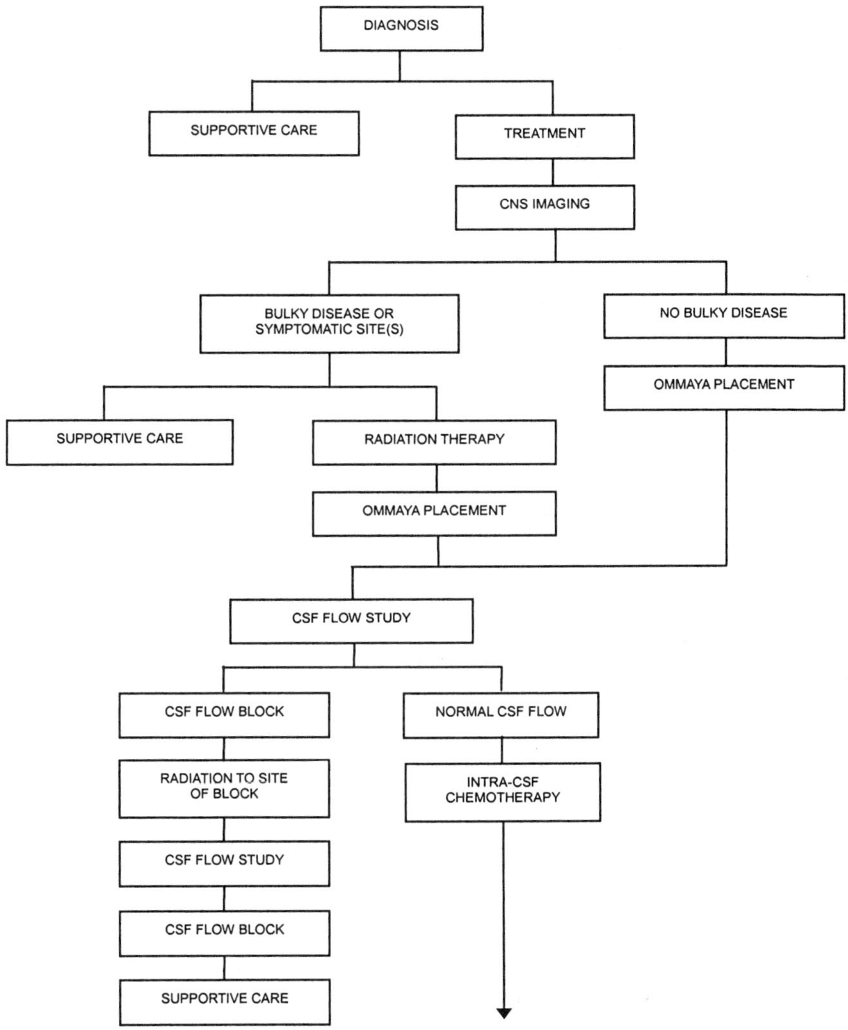

Figure 1: TREATMENT ALGORITHM OF NEOPLASTIC MENININGITIS (Continued)

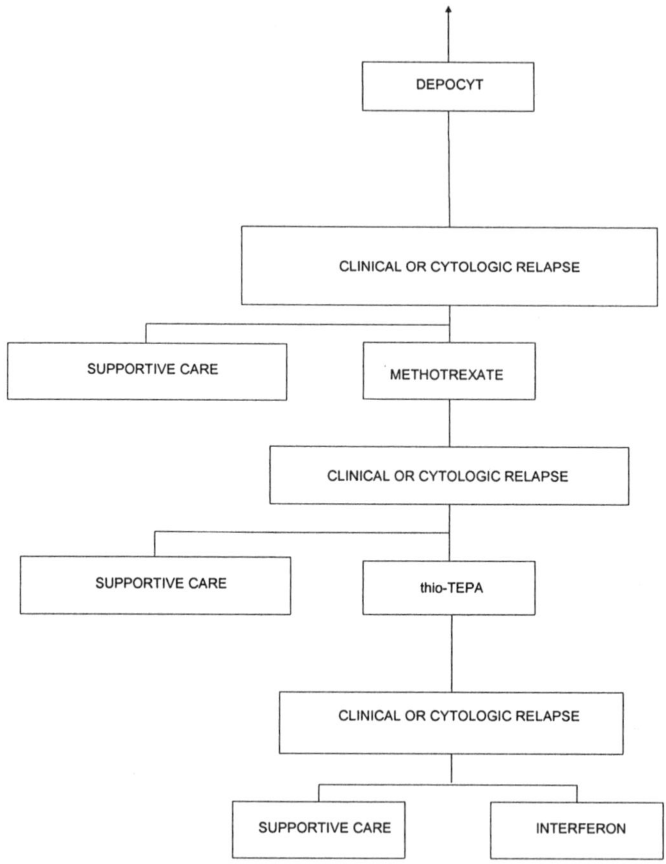

Treatment often consists of involved-field radiotherapy, systemic chemotherapy and intrathecal chemotherapy. Because meningeal dissemination most often occurs in the setting of advanced systemic tumor (in approximately 70% of all patients with neoplastic meningitis), survival after a diagnosis of meningeal carcinomatosis is usually less than six months and is in part dependent upon primary tumor histology (Table 3). [23,27] Thus, treatment is usually considered palliative rather than curative.[28-33] The exception is in childhood CNS leukemia, where durable remissions may be obtained in patients who present with CNS disease at diagnosis or who have CNS relapse after initial therapy. [23-26,34] In addition, adult patients with breast cancer or lymphoma have median survivals averaging 7-10 months, suggesting that there is a subset of patients with neoplastic meningitis who have meaningful palliation following treatment. [23,27]

Table 3: Leptomeningeal metastases: survival

	Median Survival (months)
Not treated	1.0
Treated non-responding	2.0
Primary tumor histology institutional data based on selected patients	
Melanoma	4.0
Non-small cell lung	6.0
AIDS-related lymphoma	6.0
Breast	7.5
Non-AIDS-related lymphoma	

Corticosteroids may be helpful in reducing symptoms of increased intracranial pressure although these effects are temporary. Chemotherapy may reduce symptoms when disease is treated early or if pain is the dominant symptom. Radiotherapy (Chapter 9) is useful in targeting bulky disease (subarachnoid or intraparenchymal) defined neuroradiographically, treating symptomatic regions of involvement (e.g., lumbar spine irradiation in patients with cauda equina syndrome) and treating sites of CSF flow obstruction demonstrated by either MRI or radioisotope CSF flow studies. Early recognition of neoplastic meningitis and timely treatment are important if neurologic symptoms and signs are to be reversed. In general, once neurologic deficits are established, treatment has limited impact on reversing signs resulting from neoplastic meningitis.

2. TREATMENT

Patients can present with a variety of symptoms, which may be topographically nonspecific (vomiting, headache), focal (cranial nerve palsy, paraparesis) or multifocal (encephalopathy in conjunction with cranial nerve dysfunction).[23,27] Any of these pleomorphic clinical manifestations warrant consideration of meningeal disease in patients with cancer. In general, patients present with neurologic symptoms and signs referable to three CNS domains: the cerebral hemispheres, cranial nerves or spinal cord/nerve roots.[16] Headache, nausea and vomiting, or mental status changes suggest cerebral hemisphere involvement, whereas diplopia, facial weakness, dysphagia and hearing loss are suggestive of cranial nerve involvement. Spinal cord or nerve root involvement may cause back pain only, radiculopathy, myelopathy or paraparesis.[16,23,27] Because these signs and symptoms can be vague or diffuse, clinicians must remember to consider leptomeningeal carcinomatosis in the differential diagnosis of a wide variety of clinical presentations in the cancer patient. In addition, the diagnosis is not always evident in CSF cytology or radiographic studies. Approximately 50% of patients with pathologically proven neoplastic meningitis have consistently negative antemortem CSF cytology[35], and not all patients with leptomeningeal metastasis have neuroradiographic findings consistent with neoplastic meningitis.[23,27,36,37] Thus, there is a substantial but infrequently recognized subset of patients with neoplastic meningitis who have both negative CSF cytology and negative or uninformative neuroradiographic studies. Therefore, a diagnosis of leptomeningeal carcinomatosis may be made in three clinical contexts: (1) in patients with positive CSF cytology regardless of clinical syndrome or results of neuroimaging; (2) in patients with positive neuroimaging studies (either brain or spine) consistent with leptomeningeal metastasis regardless of clinical syndrome or CSF cytology; and (3) in patients with known cancer and a clinical syndrome consistent with neoplastic meningitis in whom CSF cytology and neuraxis neuroimaging is negative.[27]

Once a diagnosis of leptomeningeal carcinomatosis is made, deciding whom to treat is a difficult problem.[28-32] Performance status and extent of systemic cancer influence outcome in patients with neoplastic meningitis. An additional consideration is the extent of the disease in the CNS.[33,38-41] The presence of epidural spinal cord compression, parenchymal brain metastases, or bulky subarachnoid nodules may identify patients who are poor candidates for intrathecal chemotherapy. Blockage of CSF flow, as demonstrated by radionuclide ventriculography, suggests cancerous adhesions even in patients with normal neuroradiography and failure of radiotherapy to restore normal CSF flow may be a poor prognostic sign.[31,42] Based on these prognostic variables, a majority of adult patients may not be candidates for aggressive neoplastic meningitis-directed therapy.

An additional difficulty is that, because progression of systemic cancer accounts for 50-60% of deaths in patients with neoplastic meningitis and treatment-related complications for another 1-5% of deaths, it is difficult to assess response rates or duration of responses for those patients with truly progressive neoplastic meningitis.[28-31,33,43,44] When treatment is initiated, the response to treatment is primarily measured by clearing of CSF cytology and secondarily by clinical improvement of neurologic signs and symptoms.[23,27,33,45] Thus, both selection of appropriate therapy and evaluation of response to that therapy can be difficult. In the following sections we outline approaches to systemic therapy, intrathecal therapy, and other measures for symptom control.

3. SYSTEMIC THERAPY

Systemic chemotherapeutic treatment of neoplastic meningitis often fails due to poor CSF penetration of nearly all chemotherapeutic agents and the difficulty in achieving significant intra-CSF drug exposures [46-57] (Table 4). Exceptions are seen with systemic high-dose intravenous methotrexate, cytarabine and thio-TEPA, all of which produce cytotoxic CSF levels and have successfully been used to treat neoplastic meningitis. Notwithstanding the theoretical limitations of systemic chemotherapy in the treatment of patients with neoplastic meningitis, several authors contend that this approach may be sufficient and obviate the need for intra-CSF chemotherapy. A provocative study by Siegal suggests that a subset of patients with neoplastic meningitis, predominantly patients with lymphoma or breast cancer, may respond to standard dose systemic chemotherapy without the inclusion of intra-CSF therapy.[58] Similar conclusions were reached by Boogerd and Fizazi, suggesting the importance of systemic chemotherapy in treating patients with neoplastic meningitis.[59,60]

Table 4. CNS penetration of chemotherapy drugs commonly used for systemic treatment of leptomeningeal tumor

Drug	CSF: Plasma Ratio (%)
Antimetabolites	
Methotrexate	3
Mercaptopurine	25
Cytarabine	20
Alkylating Agents	
Thiotepa	>90
Antimetabolites	
Topotecan	30
Irinotecan/SN-38	14/ND
Miscellaneous	
Prednisolone	<10
Dexamethasone	15
L-Asparaginase	ND

Systemic therapy provides several potential advantages in the treatment of leptomeningeal cancer. Intravenous administration allows a uniform distribution of drugs throughout the CNS and penetration of drug into the brain parenchyma and areas of bulky tumor. Furthermore, continuous intravenous infusion permits maintenance of cytotoxic CNS drug concentrations for a relatively prolonged period. As mentioned, however, most chemotherapeutic agents penetrate poorly into the CNS, and must be used in high doses to achieve therapeutic CNS concentrations. This high dose or prolonged infusion approach often results in severe systemic toxicity. The agents most commonly administered systemically for the treatment of meningeal disease are discussed below.

3.1 Methotrexate

Intravenously administered methotrexate is occasionally used in a prophylactic manner, particularly in strategies designed to decrease the risk of CNS relapse of leukemia (CNS prophylaxis or CNS preventive therapy) or when treating primary CNS lymphoma in patients without evidence of lymphomatous meningitis. In addition, systemic methotrexate may be effective in the treatment of overt CNS leukemia or lymphoma.[46] In one report comparing patients with recurrent primary CNS lymphoma complicated by lymphomatous meningitis, there was no difference in survival between treatment with high-dose methotrexate or intra-CSF methotrexate. Rather the differences between the groups related to toxicity (high-dose methotrexate was complicated by mucositis and renal insufficiency) and costs (high-dose methotrexate is expensive and usually requires patient hospitalization).[61]

Although the CSF:plasma ratio for methotrexate is only 3%,[48] cytotoxic methotrexate concentrations can be attained in the CSF using very high intravenous doses (3-8mg/m^2). Such high-dose methotrexate regimens must include both intense hydration and alkalinization of urine, and leucovorin rescue.[62] Because methotrexate is eliminated by the kidney, adequacy of renal function should be confirmed prior to therapy, and serum creatinine and methotrexate concentrations should be monitored during therapy. If methotrexate clearance is delayed, the intravenous fluid and leucovorin doses should be increased accordingly.[62] It is important to note, however, that leucovorin rescue may be ineffective when methotrexate concentrations exceed 10^{-4} mol/L.[62] In addition, because methotrexate is nephrotoxic, delayed methotrexate clearance may result in impaired renal function, with a further decrease in methotrexate clearance.[47] Acute renal failure with severely delayed methotrexate excretion is an emergency. In this situation, intravenous administration of carboxypeptidase-G2, an enzyme that cleaves methotrexate and results in a greater than ten-fold reduction of serum methotrexate concentrations within minutes of administration, may be considered.[63] Information about the availability of carboxypeptidase for emergency use can be obtained from the National Cancer Institute.

Toxicity after high-dose methotrexate occurs frequently even when renal function is adequate and proper hydration and leucovorin rescue are administered. Moderate to severe mucositis is common. Myelosuppression, hepatic toxicity, and desquamating dermatitis of the hands and feet can also occur. High-dose systemic methotrexate, especially when given in association with cranial radiation, has also been linked with neurotoxicity, manifesting as either an acute encephalopathy, which is rare, or a more common late leukoencephalopathy.[64,65]

3.2 Cytarabine

The nucleoside analog cytarabine (ara-C, cytosine arabinoside) may also be useful when administered systemically for the treatment of meningeal cancer, particularly leukemic or lymphomatous meningitis. No data is available, however, regarding the utility of high-dose cytarabine in the treatment of carcinomatous meningitis. The CSF penetration of cytarabine is approximately 20%.[56,66] Several approaches for systemic cytarabine administration have been utilized. A regimen of 3 g/m^2 administered every 12 hours demonstrated activity in patients with meningeal leukemia,[49], and a 72 hour continuous intravenous infusion of doses ≥4 g/m^2 achieved cytotoxic CSF cytarabine concentrations.[50] High-dose systemic cytarabine administration is associated with significant toxicity, with severe myelosuppression nearly universal. In addition, cerebellar dysfunction occurs in approximately 20% of patients receiving of 3 g/m^2 of cytarabine every 12 hours, especially patients older than 60 years, and requires discontinuation of therapy.[51] Nausea, vomiting, and mucositis are also common at these high doses.

3.3 Thiotepa

Thiotepa is a lipid-soluble alkylating agent that effectively crosses the blood-brain barrier. Furthermore, TEPA, an active metabolite of thiotepa, also penetrates into the CSF.[52,53] Thus, systemic administration of this agent achieves high concentrations of both parent drug and active metabolite in the CSF. Systemic thiotepa showed some activity against medulloblastoma in a pediatric phase II trial.[53] However, thiotepa causes severe bone marrow toxicity which has limited the usefulness of this agent outside the setting of dose intensive chemotherapy with stem cell rescue and cytokine support. In children with recurrent primary brain tumors, the presence of neoplastic meningitis has increasingly been recognized as a contraindication to dose intensive chemotherapy, as observed survival in such patients has been no better with high dose than conventional dose chemotherapy.

3.4 6-Mercaptopurine

The CSF penetration of 6-mercaptopurine is approximately 25%. Prolonged infusion of this drug at dose rates of 50 mg/m^2/hr achieves cytotoxic concentrations (>1 μM) in the CSF.[67] The common toxicities include reversible hepatotoxicity, myelosuppression, and mucositis.[68] Despite the relatively favorable pharmacokinetics, however, the overall activity of intravenous mercaptopurine against meningeal spread of solid tumors has been disappointing, and this approach is rarely used.[68]

3.5 Topoisomerase I inhibitors

Topotecan, a topoisomerase I inhibitor, achieves an $AUC_{csf}AUC_{plasma}$ ratio of 30% after intravenous administration.[69] In CNS tumors, topotecan administered as a 24-hour continuous infusion was not active.[70] Other studies of systemic topotecan in either primary brain tumors or in CNS metastasis from non-CNS primary tumors have shown modest activity at best. [71-73] The usefulness of intravenous topotecan against leptomeningeal carcinomatosis has not been confirmed to date.

3.6 Irinotecan

Irinotecan (CPT-11) is a prodrug of the active topoisomerase I inhibitor SN-38 that requires hepatic activation. Irinotecan itself penetrates reasonably well into the CSF, with an AUC_{csf}:AUC_{plasma} of about 14%. However, the active compound SN-38 is not detectable in CSF after intravenous irinotecan administration.[74] Three reports of irinotecan in adults with gliomas suggest limited activity for recurrent gliomas; however, none of these studies specifically treated patients with meningeal gliomatosis.[75-77] A phase II study of irinotecan in pediatric solid tumors, including tumors with leptomeningeal dissemination, is now underway in the Children's Oncology Group. This trial should help to define the usefulness of irinotecan in the treatment of leptomeningeal cancers.

4. CORTICOSTEROIDS

Prednisone (the orally administered prodrug of prednisolone) and dexamethasone, agents commonly used in the treatment of acute lymphoblastic leukemia, both penetrate into the CNS producing CSF concentrations that are equal to the plasma concentrations of free drug. However, dexamethasone is less protein bound than prednisone at equipotent doses. Therefore, dexamethasone can be considered to penetrate better into the CSF.[78] Patients receiving dexamethasone rather than prednisone for CNS preventive therapy of leukemia have a significantly lower rate of CNS relapse.[79] In some settings the infectious complications in patients receiving dexamethasone exceed those in patients receiving prednisone in an otherwise comparable chemotherapy regimen.[80] Thus, the substitution of dexamethasone for prednisone in leukemia therapy is not universal.

Dexamethasone is often used as a supportive care agent for the treatment of either chemotherapy induced nausea or edema associated with intracranial tumors. In addition, oral dexamethasone is useful to mitigate the symptoms of intrathecal (IT) chemotherapy-induced chemical meningitis. Two recent trials have demonstrated that chemical meningitis is common following intrathecal chemotherapy irrespective of the agent used and is easily managed by oral dexamethasone.[28,29]

4.1 L-asparaginase

L-asparaginase is an enzyme that hydrolyzes L-asparagine, an amino acid essential for lymphoblasts but not for normal cells. L-asparaginase does not penetrate into the CSF but may still be useful in the treatment of meningeal leukemia.[81] Following systemic administration of this agent, plasma levels of L-asparagine are depleted for a prolonged period.[82,83] Although the enzyme is not detectable in CSF, CSF L-asparagine levels are also depleted for a variable amount of time following systemic administration.[84,85]

5. INTRATHECAL THERAPY

Intrathecal chemotherapy is a form of regional therapy directed specifically against leptomeningeal cancer. IT administration of relatively small drug doses produces very high CSF drug concentration usually with minimal systemic toxicity.[86] This pharmacokinetic advantage, however, is counterbalanced by limitations that must also be considered. For example, diffusion of drug from the CSF into the brain parenchyma or tumor nodules is limited to within a few millimeters of the CSF space.[87] Thus, bulky leptomeningeal nodules may not be treated effectively with intrathecally-administered agents. In addition, drug distribution throughout the CSF compartment, especially after intralumbar dosing, may be uneven because of the slow circulation of CSF and the rapid diffusion of most intrathecally administered drugs out of the CSF. For example, drug exposure in the ventricular CSF following an intralumbar dose of methotrexate is only one-tenth of that achieved after an equivalent intraventricular dose.[48] There are also technical difficulties with IT drug administration. CSF flow is sometimes abnormal as a result of blockage by tumor.[88] In this situation, there is the concern that IT drug administration may result in unexpected toxicity if drug is not distributed throughout the CSF space. In addition, intralumbar injection is inconvenient and may be painful. Furthermore, approximately 10 % of intralumbar injections are estimated be ineffective because of leakage of the drug into the epidural space or surrounding tissues.[42]

Although systemic toxicity is uncommon after IT administration of anticancer agents, neurologic toxicity is common. In addition, inadvertent IT administration of some commonly used anticancer drugs (e.g. vincristine) is usually lethal, and IT overdose of other drugs (e.g. methotrexate) can also be fatal or life threatening.

A further disadvantage of the IT approach is the limited number of drugs that have been developed for IT use (Table 5). Methotrexate, cytarabine, hydrocortisone, and thiotepa are the only agents commonly used for direct intra-CSF administration.[23,27-31,86] A number of investigational agents are being explored including mafosfamide and 4-hydroperoxy-cyclophosphamide (derivatives of cyclophosphamide), busulfan, topotecan, diaziquinone, interferon, monoclonal antibodies, gene therapy and interleukin-2.[44,89-100] However, these agents are available only in an experimental protocol setting.

Table-5. Drugs administered by the intrathecal route

Standard agents	Investigational Agents
Methotrexate	Busulfan
Cytarabine	Mafosfamide
Hydrocortisone	Topotecan
Thiotepa	Diaziquinone
DepoCyt	4-Hydroperoxy-cyclophosphamide
	Immunotherapy
	Interferon
	Monoclonal antibody (with or without radioactive ligand)
	Interleukin-2
	Gene therapy

Some commonly used IT drug doses and schedules are listed in Tables 6 and 7. It is imperative that IT therapy only be administered by individuals familiar with the doses, schedules, and toxicities of each agent.

Table 6. Bolus intrathecal chemotherapy regimens

Drug	Induction (4 weeks)	Consolidation (4 weeks)	Maintenance
MTX[a]	10-15 mg twice weekly	10-15 mg weekly	10-15 mg monthly
Cyt	25-100 mg twice weekly	25-100 mg weekly	25-100 mg monthly
Depocyt	50 mg QOW	50 mg QOW	50 mg monthly
Thiotepa	10 mg twice weekly	10 mg weekly	10 mg monthly
Interferon	$1x10^6$ thrice weekly	$1x10^6$ weekly	$1x10^6$ monthly

QOW = every other week

Table-7. CxT intrathecal chemotherapy regimen

Drug	Induction	Consolidation	Maintenance
MTX	2 mg/day for 3-5 days, QOW x 4	2 mg/day for 3-5 days QOWx2	2 mg/day for 3-5days monthly
Cytarabine	15-25 mg/dayx3 days, weekly x 4	15-25 mg/dayx3 days QOWx2	15-25 mg/dx3days monthly
Thiotepa	10mg/dayx3days weekly x 4	10mg/dayx3 days QOWx2	10mg/dayx3days monthly

QOW = every other week
There is no CxT regimen available for Depocyt or Interferon

At present, there is no compelling data to suggest an improved response when using multiple agents versus single agent intra-CSF drug therapy. Two randomized trials in adults with carcinomatous meningitis demonstrated no survival advantage when comparing single agent (methotrexate) to polyagent (methotrexate, cytarabine and hydrocortisone) IT chemotherapy.[30,43] Furthermore, these trials suggested that polyagent IT therapy is associated with increased toxicity and less well tolerated by patients.

Because of the inconvenience and technical difficulties associated with lumbar puncture, many North American neuro-oncologists treat patients with neoplastic meningitis by the intraventricular route utilizing an intraventricular catheter and subgaleal reservoir (Ommaya reservoir). A variety of drug schedules exist and most commonly drug is administered in a bolus manner, typically twice a week.[16-19,28-31,43] Alternatively, placement of an intraventricular catheter permits the use of a concentration times time (C x T) approach based on pharmacokinetic principles.[101-107]

Few studies have compared differing intra-CSF drug schedules or drug doses in the treatment of leptomeningeal metastasis. Pharmacokinetic studies of intra-CSF drug administration in neoplastic meningitis demonstrate sustained cytotoxic lumbar and ventricular chemotherapeutic drug levels following administration by the ventricular route; however, similar studies following drug administration by the lumbar route are highly inconsistent with respect to achievement of cytotoxic ventricular chemotherapeutic drug levels.[48] Notwithstanding the pharmacokinetic advantages of intraventricular CSF drug administration as compared to intralumbar CSF drug administration, there are no studies proving that this method of administration results in improved patient survival when compared to intralumbar drug administration.

Despite the lack of conclusive evidence, many neuro-oncologists utilize a CxT method of drug delivery by the ventricular route in the hope that it will result in a lower frequency of neurotoxicity, improved tumor cell killing due to prolonged drug exposure, and better palliation and patient survival.

Whether to give intra-CSF chemotherapy concurrently with radiotherapy is problematic. The only published prospective randomized trials of neoplastic meningitis permitted both concurrent radiotherapy and intra-CSF chemotherapy, but this approach may result in an increased risk of delayed neurotoxicity as discussed below.[28,29,32]

Complications of intra-CSF drug therapy are not uncommon and may profoundly affect patients with neoplastic meningitis (Table 8).[108,109]

Table 8. Complications: intraventricular chemotherapy

	Patients	%
Meningitis	62	43
Aseptic/chemical	52	43
Bacterial (catheter infection)	9	8
Myelosuppression	21	18
Transfusion-requiring	6	5
Unidirectional catheter obstruction	5	6
Catheter misplacement	2	2
Reservoir exposure	2	2
Chemotherapy-related leukoencephalopathy	2	2
Chemotherapy-related myelopathy	1	1
1110 cycles of intraventricular chemotherapy (median 10)		
4400 Ommaya punctures (median 46)		

The placement of intraventricular catheters and subgaleal reservoirs are well known and fortunately infrequent. Misplacement of the catheter tip may be identified on post-operative plain skull films, CT or MRI and radionuclide ventriculography. Clinically significant hemorrhage is distinctly uncommon in occurrence primarily because of meticulous attention to pre-operative coagulation parameters. Infection is unfortunately a difficult problem seen at the time of intraventricular catheter placement or as a consequence of its use and occurs in up to 8% of patients. In both circumstances, skin flora, primarily *Staphylococcus epidermidis,* contaminates the system and results in iatrogenic bacterial meningitis. These infections may often be treated successfully with a combination of systemic and intraventricular antibiotics, thus preserving the intraventricular system and thereby avoiding Ommaya system removal and ultimately a re-operation. Infrequently, patients with intraventricular catheter and subgaleal reservoirs develop pressure necrosis of the skin overlying the reservoir, resulting in reservoir exposure and necessitating removal and, if clinically appropriate, replacement. Overall, serious complications requiring surgery are infrequent (6%) and most often secondary to catheter infections, Ommaya reservoir exposure or initial catheter misplacement.[108,109]

The most common complication of intraventricular catheter use relates to the toxicity of administering drugs directly into the CNS. The majority of these complications are inflammatory and transient in nature and are best characterized as aseptic chemical meningitis with fever, headache, nausea, vomiting, meningismus, photophobia and occasionally dehydration. This complication is usually easily managed in the outpatient setting with oral antipyretics, antiemetics and steroids. Direct neurotoxicity rarely occurs as a manifestation of intra-CSF drug administration which may result in either a chemotherapy-related leukoencephalopathy or myelopathy. [65,110,111] These complications may be idiosyncratic or in some instances related to total intra-CSF drug dose and delayed drug clearance. In patients with prolonged survival, the incidence of treatment-related delayed neurotoxicity manifested primarily as a leukoencephalopathy is considerably higher and may approach 30%. This delayed neurotoxicity, defined by either neuroradiographical or clinical criteria, reflects the combined effects of both radiotherapy and intra-CSF chemotherapy and appears to be an unavoidable consequence of treatment. The majority of patients treated with partial or whole brain radiotherapy develop neuroradiographic evidence of leukoencephalopathy, which fortunately is clinically apparent in only a minority. Administering intra-CSF methotrexate prior to the application of cranial irradiation may mitigate delayed neurotoxicity. The issue of timing of radiotherapy vis-à-vis methotrexate administration is more problematic in patients with neoplastic meningitis, as radiotherapy is most often utilized initially to treat symptomatic or bulky intracranial disease.

6. STANDARD AGENTS

6.1 Methotrexate

Methotrexate has been the mainstay of IT chemotherapy for over 40 years.[16-19,23,27,29,30,32,43] It is used for CNS preventive therapy in nearly all patients with acute leukemia.[112]. In addition, it is the drug most commonly used for CNS reinduction therapy in meningeal relapse of leukemia.[112-114] Because it is successful against leukemia, and there is a large body of experience with its IT administration, methotrexate is sometimes also used as "standard" therapy for the treatment of meningeal spread of solid tumors. However, the response rate of solid tumors to methotrexate is low in this setting (approximately 20%). [29,32]

Methotrexate is detectable in plasma for relatively long periods after IT dosing, but at low concentrations.[48] Although systemic toxicity is not usually a problem after an IT dose, some protocols call for administration of a single low oral Leucovorin dose after IT methotrexate. In contrast to systemic toxicity, acute or delayed neurotoxicity is relatively common after IT methotrexate. Chemical arachnoiditis, with headache, photophobia, back pain, meningismus, fever, nausea, vomiting, and CSF pleocytosis, often occurs (50% in a prospective study).[29,32] This transient aseptic meningitis has an onset on day 1-2, peaks by day 2-3 and resolves by day 5. Transient or permanent weakness or paraplegia may occur following intralumbar administration of methotrexate. This toxicity is fortunately rare and may be related to delayed clearance of methotrexate from the CSF.[110,111,115] Late neurotoxicity in the form of leukoencephalopathy may also occur, usually in patients who have received intravenous methotrexate and cranial irradiation in addition to IT methotrexate.[110,111,115]

IT methotrexate overdoses can be fatal. Immediate treatment includes ventriculolumbar perfusion to attempt to reduce methotrexate concentrations in the CNS, administration of systemic corticosteroids, and administration of systemic leucovorin.[116] In the nonhuman primate model, IT administration of carboxypeptidase-G2 immediately decreases CSF methotrexate concentrations very rapidly and prevents toxicity after experimental IT methotrexate overdose.[117] The role of carboxypeptidase-G2 in the treatment of IT methotrexate overdose in humans is unknown.

IT methotrexate therapy is often given through an Ommaya reservoir in patients with refractory meningeal disease. Administration through a reservoir produces more even drug distribution throughout the CSF compared with intralumbar administration and appears to prolong the duration of remission in CNS leukemia. [48,101,118]Use of the Ommaya reservoir also permits the administration of frequent small doses of methotrexate instead of single large doses. C x T therapy produces cytotoxic concentrations for a prolonged period while avoiding high peak drug levels. This combination may result in greater efficacy with less toxicity. [101] In this regimen, methotrexate may be administered as 2 mg per day for 3 - 5 consecutive days every other week for 4 treatment weeks (total 8 weeks), followed by administration at a decreased frequency in consolidation and maintenance phases.

Unlike systemically administered anticancer agents, IT drugs are usually given at a fixed dose, rather than body-surface area based dosing, in older children and adults. The reason for this is that, in contrast to body surface area, the CSF volume approaches adult size by the age of approximately three years. Therefore, the dose for IT methotrexate is based on patient age, with a constant dose administered to all patients over three years of age. For methotrexate, this dosing scheme both reduces toxicity in older patients and improves outcome in younger patients.[119]. Because of these seminal observations, most other IT agents are also dosed based on age rather than body size.

6.2 Cytarabine

Like methotrexate, cytarabine can be administered intrathecally to produce high CSF cytarabine concentrations with minimal systemic toxicity. Cytarabine may be given by the intralumbar route or via an Ommaya reservoir on a C x T schedule that has the same advantages as C x T methotrexate administration.[102-107] In addition, cytarabine is often combined with methotrexate and/or hydrocortisone for IT administration in children with leukemic meningitis; this is the only standard regimen for combination IT therapy. IT administration of cytarabine, like methotrexate, may produce arachnoiditis or, rarely, other forms of neurotoxicity such as seizures and paraplegia.[120] Leukoencephalopathy and other chronic neurotoxicities, however, have not been described commonly with IT cytarabine.

6.3 Liposomal Cytarabine

A liposomal encapsulated form of cytarabine (DepoCyt™) has been shown to be an active agent with potential advantages compared to free cytarabine or methotrexate.[28,29,32,122] These advantages include once every two-week drug administration whether the intraventricular or intralumbar route is used. Two randomized trials in adults compared liposomal cytarabine to methotrexate (in patients with carcinomatous meningitis) or free cytarabine (in patients with lymphomatous meningitis).[28,29] In both trials, the response rate was better, the time to neurologic disease progression was delayed, and death due to neoplastic meningitis was reduced in the liposomal cytarabine cohort. No difference in survival between the treatment arms was seen in either trial, but quality of life was improved in the liposomal cytarabine cohort. Because of the convenience of once every two weeks administration in addition to the modest merits mentioned above, liposomal cytarabine is increasingly being considered as first-line therapy for either carcinomatous or lymphomatous meningitis. Insufficient data exists regarding liposomal cytarabine's effectiveness for leukemic meningitis, though an on-going Phase 1 trial in pediatric neoplastic meningitis may generate some conclusions. Importantly, because of a high incidence of chemical meningitis when this agent is administered without corticosteroids, oral dexamethasone at a dose of 2 – 4 mg by mouth twice per day for 5 days should be utilized whenever liposomal cytarabine is administered regardless of delivery route.

6.4 Thiotepa

IT administration of thiotepa, in contrast to systemic administration of the same agent, is well tolerated although it may be associated with myelosuppression.[31] The active metabolite TEPA, however, is not detected in CSF after IT administration. In addition, because the drug is highly lipid soluble unlike most other intrathecally administered agents, thiotepa diffuses rapidly out of the CSF.[121] Thus, the usual pharmacokinetic advantages of IT drug administration may be less prominent for thiotepa than for some other drugs. Nonetheless, IT thiotepa has been shown in one of four randomized trials in adults with neoplastic meningitis to be as effective as methotrexate. Thiotepa may also be administered on a C x T schedule. No survival benefit has been demonstrated when comparing thiotepa to methotrexate in the treatment of neoplastic meningitis in adult carcinomatous meningitis.[31]

7. INVESTIGATIONAL AGENTS

7.1 Mafosfamide

Mafosfamide is a preactivated derivative of cyclophosphamide that does not require hepatic metabolism to have antitumor activity. This agent has demonstrated activity in phase I trials against meningeal leukemia and leptomeningeal dissemination of brain tumors.[92,99] It is currently undergoing further study in an adult Phase 1 trial and in the Pediatric Brain Tumor Consortium to determine its efficacy in adult carcinomatous meningitis and in preventing leptomeningeal recurrence of primary brain tumors in infants, respectively.[93]

7.2 Topotecan

IT administration of the topoisomerase I poison topotecan was studied in a recent phase I trial in children.[123] Arachnoiditis was the dose-limiting toxicity, and the maximum tolerated dose was 0.4 mg. Several patients with leptomeningeal spread of solid tumors demonstrated responses or prolonged stable disease. A phase II trial of IT topotecan in children with neoplastic meningitis is in progress in the Children's Oncology Group as is a Phase 1 trial in adults with carcinomatous meningitis.

7.3 Monoclonal antibodies

Monoclonal antibody therapy directed at meningeal metastasis is a relatively new approach that theoretically has the advantage of selectively targeting malignant cells that express specific antigens while sparing normal tissues that do not share these epitopes. Most studies have utilized ^{131}I linked to an antibody of interest (so- called radioimmunoconjugates) in the particular tumor being studied. Toxicity, particularly systemic myelosuppression, and the need to have an appropriate antibody limit this approach at present although it remains under exploration.[91,94-98,100]

8. SYMPTOMATIC THERAPY

A variety of medical therapies are utilized in the care of patients with leptomeningeal metastasis irrespective of whether the patient is offered aggressive neoplastic meningitis-directed therapy. A minority of patients will manifest seizures as a consequence of neoplastic meningitis and the use of non-sedating anticonvulsant drugs is appropriate for this group of patients. Patients with difficult to control pain may be managed with narcotics or, in the instance of neuropathic pain, either anticonvulsant drug or tricyclic antidepressant drug therapy. Depression is a very common symptom in patients with cancer and is often neglected or not recognized. Early recognition and initiation of antidepressants in symptomatic patients is recognized to improve quality of life and benefit both patients and families. In addition, antidepressants, especially tricyclic agents, are also useful for chronic insomnia. Corticosteroids are most useful to control vasogenic edema secondary to parenchymal brain or epidural metastases but have very limited use in the management of neoplastic meningitis-related neurologic symptoms. Steroids may be useful in patients with raised intracranial pressure or in patients with chronic nausea or vomiting. Similarly, nausea or vomiting may be managed by anti-emetics. Concurrent steroids, megestrol acetate or cannabinols may mitigate weight loss and cancer-related anorexia. Finally, decreased attention and somnolence, common side effects of whole brain irradiation and chemotherapy, may be improved modestly by the use of psychostimulants such as dextroamphetamine or modafinil.

9. CONCLUSIONS

Neoplastic meningitis is a complicated disease for a variety of reasons. Not all patients necessarily warrant aggressive CNS-directed therapy, yet few guidelines exist permitting appropriate choice of therapy. In general, only pain-related neurologic symptoms improve with treatment. Neurologic signs such as confusion, cranial nerve deficit(s), ataxia and segmental weakness minimally improve or stabilize with successful treatment. The majority of patients die due to progressive systemic disease occurring either in isolation or in combination with progressive neoplastic meningitis. Notwithstanding aggressive treatment, survival ranges only from 2-10 months depending upon tumor histology, and in adult neoplastic meningitis, therapy is considered palliative rather than curative. However, specific tumor histologies may have different responses to therapy. For example, the consensus is that breast cancer is inherently more chemosensitive than non-small cell lung cancer or melanoma, and therefore, survival following chemotherapy is likely to be better. This observation has been substantiated in patients with systemic metastases though comparable data regarding CNS metastases, and in particular neoplastic meningitis, is meager.[32,59,60]

Supportive comfort care (radiotherapy to symptomatic disease, antiemetics, and narcotics) rather than aggressive therapy may reasonably be offered to a majority of adults with neoplastic meningitis. Palliative therapy of neoplastic meningitis often affords the patient protection from further neurological deterioration and consequently an improved neurologic quality of life. No studies to date have attempted an economic assessment of the treatment of neoplastic meningitis and therefore no information is available regarding a cost-benefit analysis as has been performed for other cancer directed therapies.

A number of challenges remain in the treatment of neoplastic meningitis. Treatment failure may result from (1) *de novo* or acquired drug resistance; (2) incomplete distribution of drug within CSF spaces; (3) inability to achieve adequate CSF drug levels; (4) failure to control primary non-CNS tumor; (5) toxicity, both neurologic and systemic toxicity of regional chemotherapy; (6) concurrent CNS metastatic disease (parenchymal brain, dural and epidural spinal cord metastases); and (7) inability of patients to tolerate treatment.[28,29,32,38-41,48,124] Each of these challenges must be overcome to make substantial improvements in the therapy of leptomeningeal carcinomatosis.

REFERENCES

1. Evans A, Gilbert E, Zandstra R. The increasing incidence of central nervous system leukemia in children. Cancer 1970; 26:404-407.
2. Posner J, Chernik N. Intracranial metastases from systemic cancer. Advances in Neurology 1978; 19:579-592.
3. Boyle R, Thomas M, Adams J. Diffuse involvement of the leptomeninges by tumour- a clincial and pathological study of 63 cases. Postgraduate Med J 1980; 56:149-158.
4. Whelan HT, Sung JH, Mastri AR. Diffuse leptomeningeal gliomatosis: Report of three cases. Clin Neuropathol 1987; 6:164-168.
5. Civitello LA, Packer RJ, Rorke LB, et al. Leptomeningeal dissemination of low-grade gliomas in childhood. Neurology 1988; 38:562-566.
6. Davila G, Duyckaerts C, Lazareth JP, et al. Diffuse primary leptomeningeal gliomatosis. J Neurooncol 1993; 15:45-49.
7. Bailey P, Robitaille Y. Primary diffuse leptomeningeal gliomatosis. Can J Neurol Sci 1985; 12:278-281.
8. Ausman J, Shrontz C, Chason J, et al. Aggressive choroid plexus papilloma. Surg Neurol 1984; 22:472-476.
9. Deutsch M. The impact of myelography on the treatment results for medulloblastoma. Int J Rad Oncol Biol Phys 1984; 10:999-1003.
10. Jennings MT, Slatkin N, D'Angelo M, et al. Neoplastic meningitis as the presentation of occult primitive neuroectodermal tumors. J Child Neurol 1993; 8:306-312.

11. Ross G, Rubenstein L. Lack of histopathological correlation of malignant ependymomas with postoperative survival. J Neurosurg 1989; 70:31-36.
12. Trigg M, Makuch R, Glaubiger D. Actuarial risk of isolated cns involvement in Ewing's sarcoma following prophylactic cranial irradiation and methotrexate. Int J Radiatr Oncol Biol Phys 1985; 11:699-702.
13. Jenkin R, Simpson W, Keen C. Pineal and suprasellar germinomas: Results of treatment. J Neurosurg 1978; 48:99-107.
14. Goldwein J, Corn B, Findlay J, et al. Is craniospinal irradiation required to cure children with malignant (anaplastic) intracranial ependymomas? Cancer 1991; 67:2766-2771.
15. Olson M, Chernik N, Posner J. Infiltration of the leptomeninges by systemic cancer: A clinical and pathologic study. Arch Neurol 1974; 30:122-137.
16. Wasserstrom W, Glass J, Posner J. Diagnosis and treatment of leptomeningeal metastases from solid tumors: Experience with 90 patients. Cancer 1982; 49:759-772.
17. Little J, Dale A, Okazaki H. Meningeal carcinomatosis: Clinical manifestations. Arch Neurol 1974; 30:138-143.
18. Theodore W, Gendelman S. Meningeal carcinomatosis. Arch Neurol 1981; 38:696-699.
19. Kaplan JG, DeSouza TG, Farkash A, et al. Leptomeningeal metastases: Comparison of clinical features and laboratory data of solid tumors, lymphomas and leukemias. J Neurooncol 1990; 9:225-229.
20. Bigner S, Johnston W. The cytopathology of cerebrospinal fluid. Acta Cytologica 1981; 25:461-477.
21. Kokkoris C. Leptomeningeal carcinomatosis: How does cancer reach the pia-arachnoid? Cancer 1983; 51:154-160.
22. Gonzalez-Vitale J, Garcia-Bunuel R. Meningeal carcinomatosis. Cancer 1976; 37:2906-2911.
23. DeAngelis LM. Current diagnosis and treatment of leptomeningeal metastasis. J Neurooncol 1998; 38:245-252.
24. Gelber R, Sallan S, Cohen H, et al. Central nervous system treatment in childhood acute lymphoblastic leukemia. Cancer 1993; 72:261-270.
25. Ribeiro R, Rivera G, Hudson M, et al. An intensive re-treatment protocol for children with an isolated cns relapse of acute lymphoblastic leukemia. J Clin Oncol 1995; 13:333-358.
26. Steinherz P. Cns leukemia: Problem of diagnosis, outcome, and treatment. J Clin Oncol 1995; 13:310-313.
27. Chamberlain M, Kormanik P. Neoplastic meningitis: A guide to diagnosis and treatment. CNS Drugs 1998; 10:25-41.
28. Glantz MJ, Jaeckle KA, Chamberlain MC, et al. A randomized controlled trial comparing intrathecal sustained-release cytarabine (depocyt) to intrathecal methotrexate in patients with neoplastic meningitis from solid tumors. Clin Cancer Res 1999; 5:3394-3402.
29. Glantz M, Chamberlain M, Shapiro W, et al. A randomized trial of a slow-release formulation of cytarabine for the treatment of lymphomatous meningitis. J Clin Oncol 1999; 17:3110-3116.
30. Hitchins R, Bell D, Woods R, et al. A prospective randomized trial of single-agent versus combination therapy in meningeal carcinomatosis. J Clin Oncol 1987; 5:1655-1662.
31. Grossman SA, Finkelstein DM, Ruckdeschel JC, et al. Randomized prospective comparison of intraventricular methotrexate and thiotepa in patients with previously untreated neoplastic meningitis. Eastern cooperative oncology group. J Clin Oncol 1993; 11:561-569.
32. Jaeckle KA, Phuphanich S, Bent MJ, et al. Intrathecal treatment of neoplastic meningitis due to breast cancer with a slow-release formulation of cytarabine. Br J Cancer 2001; 84:157-163.
33. Balm M, Hammack J. Leptomeningeal carcinomatosis. Arch Neurol 1996; 53: 626-632.

34. Grossman S, Moynihan T. Neurologic complications of systemic cancer: Neoplastic meningitis. Neurol Clin 1991; 9:843-856.
35. Glass J, Melamed M, Chernik N, et al. Malignant cells in cerebrospinal fluid: The meaning of a positive CSF cytology. Neurology 1979; 29:1369-1375.
36. Chamberlain M, Sandy A, Press G. Leptomeningeal metastasis: A comparison of gadolinium-enhanced MR and contrast-enhanced ct of the brain. Neurology 1990; 40:435-438.
37. Chamberlain M. Comparative spine imaging in leptomeningeal metastases. J Neurooncol 1995; 23:233-238.
38. Glantz M, Hall W, Cole B, et al. Diagnosis, management, and survival of patients with leptomeningeal cancer based on cerebrospinal fluid-flow studies. Cancer 1995; 75:2919-2931.
39. Chamberlain M, Kormanik P. Prognostic significance of ^{111}indium-dtpa CSF flow studies. Neurology 1996; 46:1674-1677.
40. Chamberlain M, Kormanik P. Prognostic significance of co-existent bulky metastatic CNS disease in patients with leptomeningeal metastases. Arch Neurol 1997; 54:1364-1368.
41. Grossman S, Trump D, Chen D, et al. Cerebrospinal fluid flow abnormalities in patients with neoplastic meningitis. Am J Med 1982; 73:641-647.
42. Larson S, Schall G, DiChiro G. The influence of previous lumbar puncture and pneumoencephalography on the incidence of unsuccessful radioisotope cisternography. J Nuclear Med 1971; 12:555-557.
43. Giannone L, Greco F, Hainsworth J. Combination intraventricular therapy for meningeal neoplasia. J Clin Oncol 1986; 4:68-73.
44. Chamberlain M. Alpha-interferon in the treatment of neoplastic meningitis. 2002. In Press
45. Glantz M, Chamberlain M, Walters B. Diagnosis and outcome measures for neoplastic meningitis: A review of the literature and clinical experience. Neurosurgery Focus 1998; 4:Article 4.
46. Balis F, Savitch J, Bleyer W, et al. Remission induction of meningeal leukemia with high-dose intravenous methotrexate. J Clin Oncol 1985; 3:485-489.
47. Balis F, Holcenberg J, Blaney S. General prinicples of chemotherapy. In: Pizzo P, Poplack D, eds. Principles and practice of pediatric oncology. Philadelphia, PA: Lippincott, Williams, and Wilkins; 2002:237-308.
48. Shapiro W, Young D, Mehta B. Methotrexate: Distribution in cerebrospinal fluid after intravenous, ventricular, and lumbar injections. New Engl J Med 1975; 293:161-166.
49. Frick J, Rich P, Hansen R, et al. Successful treatment of meningeal leukemia using systemic high-dose cytosine arabinoside. J Clin Oncol 1984; 2:365-368.
50. Donehower R, Karp J, Burke P. Pharmacology and toxicity of high-dose cytarabine by 72-hour continuous infusion. Cancer Treat Rep 1986; 70:1059-1065.
51. Nand S, Messmore H, Patel R, et al. Neurotoxicity associated with systemic high-dose cytosine arabinoside. J Clin Oncol 1986; 4:571-575.
52. Heideman R, Cole D, Balis F, et al. Phase I and pharmacokinetic evaluation of thiotepa in the cerebrospinal fluid and plasma of pediatric patients: Evidence for dose-dependent plasma clearance of thiotepa. Cancer Res 1989; 49:736-741.
53. Heideman R, Packer R, Reaman G, et al. A phase II evaluation of thiotepa in central nervous system malignancies. Cancer 1992; 72:271-275.
54. Slevin M, Piall E, Aherne G, et al. Effect of dose and schedule on pharmacokinetics of high-dose cytosine arabinoside in plasma and cerebrospinal fluid. J Clin Oncol 1983; 1:546-551.
55. Lopez J, Nassif E, Vannicola P, et al. Central nervous system pharmacokinetics of high-dose cytosine arabinoside. J Neurooncol 1985; 3:119-124.
56. Ackland S, Schilsky R. High-dose methotrexate: A critical reappraisal. J Clin Oncol 1987; 5:2017-2031.
57. Balis FM, Poplack DG. Central nervous system pharmacology of antileukemic drugs. Am J

Pediatr Hematol Oncol 1989; 11:74-86.
58. Siegal T. Leptomeningeal metastases: Rationale for systemic chemotherapy or what is the role of intra-csf-chemotherapy? J Neurooncol 1998; 38:151-157.
59. Boogerd W, Hart AA, van, et al. Meningeal carcinomatosis in breast cancer. Prognostic factors and influence of treatment. Cancer 1991; 67:1685-1695.
60. Fizazi K, Asselain B, Vincent-Salomon A, et al. Meningeal carcinomatosis in patients with breast carcinoma. Cancer 1996; 77:1315-1323.
61. Chamberlain M, Kormanik P, Glantz M. Recurrent primary central nervous system lymphoma complicated by lymphomatous meningitis. Oncol Rep 1998; 5:521-523.
62. Pinedo H, Zaharko D, Bull J, et al. The reversal of methotrexate cytotoxicity to mouse bone marrow cells by leucovorin and nucleosides. Cancer Res 1976; 36:4418-4424.
63. Widemann B, Hetherington M, Smithson W, et al. Carboxypeptidase-g2 as a rescue agent following methotrexate induced renal failure or intrathecal methotrexate overdose. Proc Am Assoc Cancer Res 1995; 36:1384.
64. Walker R, Allen J, Rosen G, et al. Transient cerebral dysfunction secondary to high-dose methotrexate. J Clin Oncol 1986; 4:1845-1950.
65. Bleyer W. Neurologic sequelae of methotrexate and ionizing radiation: A new classification. Cancer Treat Rep 1981; 65:89-98.
66. Slevin M, Piall E, Aherne G, et al. The pharmacokinetics of cytosine arabinoside in the plasma and cerebrospinal fluid during conventional and high-dose therapy. Med Pediatr Oncol 1982; 1:157-168.
67. Zimm S, Ettinger L, Holcenberg J, et al. Phase i and clinical pharmacological study of 6-mercaptopurine administered as a prolonged intravenous infusion. Cancer Res 1985; 45:1869-1873.
68. Adamson P, Zimm S, Ragab A, et al. A phase ii trial of continuous-infusion 6-mercaptopurine for childhood solid tumors. Cancer Chemother Pharmacol 1990; 26:343-344.
69. Blaney S, Cole D, Balis F, et al. Plasma and cerebrospinal fluid pharmacokinetic study of topotecan in nonhuman primates. Cancer Res 1993; 53:725-727.
70. Blaney SM, Phillips PC, Packer RJ, et al. Phase ii evaluation of topotecan for pediatric central nervous system tumors. Cancer 1996; 78:527-531.
71. Friedman HS, Kerby T, Fields S, et al. Topotecan treatment of adults with primary malignant glioma. The brain tumor center at duke. Cancer 1999; 85:1160-1165.
72. Macdonald D, Cairncross G, Stewart D, et al. Phase ii study of topotecan in patients with recurrent malignant glioma. National clinical institute of Canada Clinical Trials Group. Ann Oncol 1996; 7:205-207.
73. Oberhoff C, Kieback DG, Wurstlein R, et al. Topotecan chemotherapy in patients with breast cancer and brain metastases: Results of a pilot study. Onkologie 2001; 24:256-260.
74. Blaney SM, Takimoto C, Murry DJ, et al. Plasma and cerebrospinal fluid pharmacokinetics of 9-aminocamptothecin (9-ac), irinotecan (cpt-11), and sn-38 in nonhuman primates. Cancer Chemother Pharmacol 1998; 41:464-468.
75. Friedman HS, Petros WP, Friedman AH, et al. Irinotecan therapy in adults with recurrent or progressive malignant glioma. J Clin Oncol 1999; 17:1516-1525.
76. Chamberlain M. Salvage chemotherapy with cpt-11 for recurrent glioblastoma multiforme. Journal of Neuro-Oncology 2002 (In Press).
77. Chamberlain M. Salvage chemotherapy with cpt-11 for oligodendroglioma. J Neurooncol 2002 (In Press).
78. Balis F, Lester C, Chrousos G, et al. Differences in cerebrospinal fluid penetration of corticosteroids: Possible relationship to the prevention of meningeal leukemia. J Clin Oncol 1987; 5:202-207.
79. Jones B, Freeman AI, Shuster JJ, et al. Lower incidence of meningeal leukemia when

prednisone is replaced by dexamethasone in the treatment of acute lymphocytic leukemia. Med Pediatr Oncol 1991; 19:269-275.
80. Hurwitz CA, Silverman LB, Schorin MA, et al. Substituting dexamethasone for prednisone complicates remission induction in children with acute lymphoblastic leukemia. Cancer 2000; 88:1964-1969.
81. Tallal L, Tan C, Oettgen H, et al. E. Coli l-asparaginase in the treatment of leukemia and solid tumors in 131 children. Cancer 1970; 25:306-320.
82. Capizzi R, Bertino J, Skeel R, et al. L-asparaginase: Clinical, biochemical, pharmacological, and immunological studies. Ann Int Med 1971; 74:893-901.
83. Ho D, Brown N, Yen A, et al. Clinical pharmacology of polyethylene glycol l-asparaginase. Drug Metab Dispos 1986; 14:349-352.
84. Berg S, Balis F, McCully C, et al. Pharmacokinetics of peg-l-asparaginase and plasma and cerebrospinal fluid l-asparagine concentrations in the rhesus monkey. Cancer Chemother Pharmacol 1993; 32:310-314.
85. Riccardi R, Holcenberg J, Glaubiger D, et al. L-asparaginase pharmacokinetics and asparagine levels in cerebrospinal fluid of rhesus monkeys and humans. Cancer Res 1981; 41:4554-4558.
86. Collins J. Pharmacokinetics of intraventricular admininstration. J Neuro-Oncol. 1983; 1:283-291.
87. Blasberg R, Patlak C, Shapiro W. Distribution of methotrexate in the cerebrospinal fluid and brain after intraventricular administration. Cancer Treat Rep 1977; 61:633-641.
88. Chamberlain MC, Corey BJ. Leptomeningeal metastases: 111indium-dtpa CSF flow studies. Neurology 1991; 41:1765-1769.
89. Arndt C, Colvin O, Balis F, et al. Intrathecal administration of 4-hydroperoxycyclophosphamide in rhesus monkeys. Cancer Res 1987; 47:5932-5934.
90. Berg SL, Balis FM, Zimm S, et al. Phase i/ii trial and pharmacokinetics of intrathecal diaziquone in refractory meningeal malignancies. J Clin Oncol 1992; 10:143-148.
91. Bigner DD, Brown M, Coleman RE, et al. Phase i studies of treatment of malignant gliomas and neoplastic meningitis with 131i-radiolabeled monoclonal antibodies anti-tenascin 81c6 and anti-chondroitin proteoglycan sulfate me1-14 f (ab')2--a preliminary report. J Neurooncol 1995; 24:109-122.
92. Blaney S, Balis F, Murphy R, et al. A phase i study of intrathecal mafosfamide in patients with refractory meningeal malignancy. Proc Am Soc Clin Oncol 1992; 11:274.
93. Blaney S, Horowitz M, Kun L, et al. A new approach to the treatment of infants with CNS tumors. Society Neuro-Oncology. Chicago, IL; 2000
94. Brown MT, Coleman RE, Friedman AH, et al. Intrathecal 131i-labeled antitenascin monoclonal antibody 81c6 treatment of patients with leptomeningeal neoplasms or primary brain tumor resection cavities with subarachnoid communication: Phase I trial results. Clin Cancer Res 1996; 2:963-972.
95. Hall WA, Fodstad O. Immunotoxins and central nervous system neoplasia. J Neurosurg 1992; 76:1-12.
96. Kemshead JT, Hopkins KI, Chandler CL. Treatment of diffuse leptomeningeal malignancy by intrathecal injection of 131i radioimmunoconjugates. Recent Results Cancer Res 1996; 141:145-158.
97. Kemshead JT, Hopkins K, Pizer B, et al. Dose escalation with repeated intrathecal injections of 131i-labelled mabs for the treatment of central nervous system malignancies. Br J Cancer 1998; 77:2324-2330.
98. Moseley RP, Papanastassiou V, Zalutsky MR, et al. Immunoreactivity, pharmacokinetics and bone marrow dosimetry of intrathecal radioimmunoconjugates. Int J Cancer 1992; 52:38-43.

99. Slavc I, Schuller E, Czech T, et al. Intrathecal mafosfamide therapy for pediatric brain tumors with meningeal dissemination. J Neurooncol 1998; 38:213-218.
100. Youle RJ. Immunotoxins for central nervous system malignancy. Semin Cancer Biol 1996; 7:65-70.
101. Bleyer W, Poplack D, Simon R. "concentration x time" methotrexate via a subcutaneous reservoir: A less toxic regimen for intraventricular chemotherapy of central nervous system neoplasms. Blood 1978; 51:835-842.
102. Chamberlain M, Dirr L. Involved field radiotherapy and intra-Ommaya methotrexate/ara-c in patients with aids-related lymphomatous meningitis. J Clin Oncol 1993; 11:1978-1984.
103. Chamberlain M, Kormanik P. Leptomeningeal metastases due to melanoma: Combined modality therapy. Int J. Oncol 1996; 9:505-510.
104. Chamberlain M, Kormanik P. Carcinomatous meningitis secondary to breast cancer: Combined modality therapy. J Neurooncol 1997; 35:55-64.
105. Chamberlain M, Kormanik P. Carcinomatous meningitis secondary to non-small cell lung cancer: Combined modality therapy. Arch Neurol 1998; 55:506-512.
106. Chamberlain M, Kormanik P. Non-aids related lymphomatous meningitis: Combined modality therapy. Neurology 1997; 49:1728-1731.
107. Chamberlain M, Kormanik P. Lymphomatous meningitis in immunocompromised patients: Combined modality therapy. Oncol Rep 1998; 5:521-525.
108. Chamberlain M, Kormanik P. Complications associated with intraventricular chemotherapy in patients with leptomeningeal metastases. J Neurosurg 1997; 87:694-699.
109. Lishner M, Perrin RG, Feld R, et al. Complications associated with Ommaya reservoirs in patients with cancer. The Princess Margaret Hospital experience and a review of the literature. Arch Intern Med 1990; 150:173-176.
110. Price R. Therapy related central nervous system diseases in children with acute lymphocytic leukemia. In: Mastrangelo R, Poplack D, Riccardi R, eds. Central nervous system leukemia. Boston: Martinus Nijhoff Publishers; 1983:71-81.
111. Ochs J. Neurotoxicity due to central nervous system therapy for childhood leukemia. Am J Ped Hematol-Oncol 1989; 11:93-105.
112. Pochedly C. Prevention of meningeal leukemia. Review of 20 years of research and current recommendations. Hematol Oncol Clin North Am 1990; 4:951-969.
113. Whiteside J, Philips F, Dargeon H, et al. Intrathecal amethopterin in neurological manifestations of leukemia. Arch Int Med 1958; 101:279-285.
114. Sullivan M, Vietti T, Fernbach D, et al. Clinical investigations in the treatment of meningeal leukemia: Radiation therapy regimens vs. Conventional intrathecal methotrexate. Blood 1969; 34:301-319.
115. Bleyer W, Drake J, Chabner B. Neurotoxicity and elevated cerebrospinal fluid methotrexate concentration in meningeal leukemia. New Engl J Med 1973; 289:770-773.
116. Addegio J, Ridgway D, Bleyer W. The acute management of intrathecal methotrexate overdose: Pharmacologic rationale and guidelines. J Pediatr 1981; 98:825-828.
117. Adamson PC, Balis FM, McCully CL, et al. Rescue of experimental intrathecal methotrexate overdose with carboxypeptidase-g2. J Clin Oncol 1991; 9:670-674.
118. Bleyer W, Poplack D. Intraventricular versus intralumbar methotrexate for central nervous-system leukemia: Prolonged remission with the Ommaya reservoir. Med Pediatr Oncol 1979; 6:207-213.
119. Bleyer W, Coccia P, Sather H, et al. Reduction in the incidence of central nervous system leukemia with a pharmacokinetically derived intrathecal methotrexate dosage regimen. J Clin Oncol 1983; 1:317-325.
120. Saiki J, Thompson S, Smith F, et al. Paraplegia following intrathecal chemotherapy. Cancer 1972; 29:370-374.

121. Strong J, Collins J, Lester C, et al. Pharmacokinetics of intraventricular and intravenous n,n',n"-triethylenethiophosphoramide (thiotepa) in rhesus monkeys and humans. Cancer Res 1986; 46:6101-6104.
122. Bleyer WA. Intrathecal depot cytarabine therapy: A welcome addition to the therapeutic armamentarium. Clin Cancer Res 1999; 5:3349-3351.
123. Blaney SM, Heideman R, Berg S, et al. Phase I clinical trial of intrathecal topotecan in patients with neoplastic meningitis. Submitted.
124. Dedrick R, Zaharko D, Bender R, et al. Pharmacokinetic considerations on resistance to anticancer drugs. Cancer Chemother Rep 1975; 59:795-804.

Chapter 9

RADIATION THERAPY FOR LEPTOMENINGEAL CANCER

Minesh Mehta, M.D. and Kristin Bradley, M.D.
University of Wisconsin Medical School, Madison, WI. 53792

Abstract: Radiotherapy has multiple roles in the treatment of leptomeningeal cancer. While it is uncommon for patients to experience regression of neurologic deficits due to leptomeningeal cancer, focal radiotherapy often provides significant palliation of pain, increased intracranial pressure and other focal symptoms. Focal radiotherapy may also be used to eliminate blockages of cerebrospinal fluid (CSF) and allow for safe administration of intrathecal chemotherapy. Craniospinal irradiation (CSI) is most often used as prophylaxis for patients at high risk of leptomeningeal tumor dissemination, but may result in symptom palliation and prolonged disease control for patients with active leptomeningeal tumor.

Key words: Radiotherapy; craniospinal irradiation; prophylaxis; cerebrospinal fluid block; whole brain radiotherapy

1. INTRODUCTION

Leptomeningeal carcinomatosis occurs in approximately 5% of patients with cancer.[1] The frequency of diagnosis is increasing as cancer patients live longer and neuro-imaging technology improves. Without treatment, the median survival is four to six weeks.[2] The specific approach to treatment depends on the tumor type and burden, the patient's symptoms and overall performance status. Surgical management and chemotherapeutic treatment of leptomeningeal cancer have been addressed in previous chapters. Radiation therapy is also used in some patients to treat leptomeningeal cancer. Craniospinal irradiation (CSI), focal external beam radiation, and investigational radiation techniques will be discussed in this chapter. The primary rationale for considering radiotherapy is two-fold: first, several patients present with significant symptoms such as cranial nerve palsies, sphincter dysfunction, limited ambulation, pain, obstructive hydrocephalus, etc., which benefit from palliative radiation; second, approximately one-half of all patients with leptomeningeal disease die as a direct consequence of compartmental progression of their disease, as opposed to systemic progression, suggesting that control of disease within the cerebrospinal fluid (CSF) compartment holds some potential for improving survival, albeit modestly.[3-5]

2. CRANIOSPINAL RADIATION

This technique treats the entire craniospinal axis and frequently is utilized with a high rate of success in other malignant diseases of the craniospinal axis, such as medulloblastoma and central nervous system (CNS) germinoma. Because of the compartmental nature of leptomeningeal carcinomatosis, craniospinal irradiation is occasionally used in the treatment of this disease process. It involves a technically complex set-up of two opposed lateral brain fields and one or two posterior spine fields (depending on the patient's height) to treat the entire craniospinal axis homogeneously without one region receiving too high or too low of a dose. The following diagram demonstrates how a craniospinal set-up is often planned.[6]

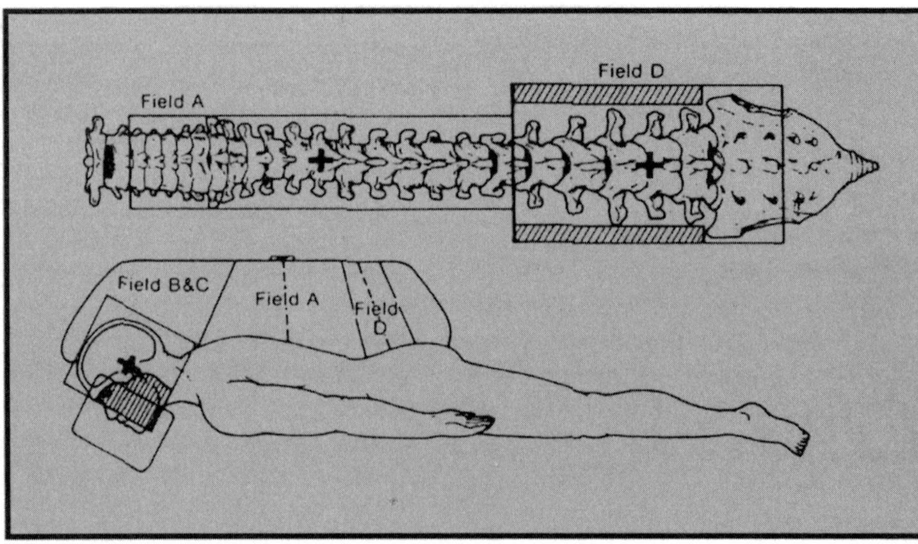

The brain and spine photon fields are matched to each other via two general approaches: 1) gapping, and 2) divergence matching. Gapping involves either positioning of the beams so that the divergent edges intersect at a depth, or directly abutting the beams so they intersect at a zero depth. This technique is referred to as "gapping" since it results in a gap on the patient's skin. Divergence matching involves positioning the beams so that their respectively divergent field surfaces are parallel and adjacent to one another at the time of treatment.[7]

Different institutions use a variety of techniques. In one commonly employed technique, the patient lies prone on the treatment table or couch. The posterior spine field is set up to treat the entire thecal sac and the superior border of the spine field is demarcated on the patient's neck. The brain is treated with opposed lateral fields. These cranial fields are set up so that their inferior borders match the longitudinal divergence of the edge of the superior spine port. This is accomplished by rotating the treatment machine's collimator of the brain field. By rotating the treatment couch, the transverse superior edge of the spine field is made parallel to the inferior divergent edge of the brain port. The two angles of rotation of the collimator and the couch are given by the formulas:

$$\theta \text{ (collimator)} = \tan^{-1} [\text{spine length} / 2 \times \text{SSD}]$$
$$\theta \text{ (couch)} = \tan^{-1} [\text{brain length} / 2 \times \text{SAD}]$$

This setup is demonstrated in the following diagram.[8]

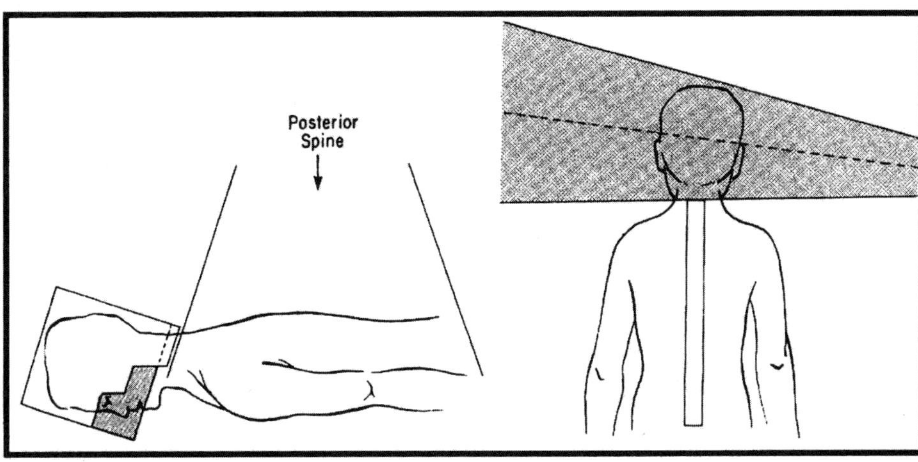

The junction line between the cranial and spinal fields is moved down on the neck one centimeter on predetermined treatment days in order to minimize hot spots. The daily radiation fraction size is generally small (1.2-1.8 Gy) with the total dose dependent on the tumor type and tumor load.

Boosts are given to areas at highest risk for relapse, such as the primary site or regions with large tumor burden.

The median survival of patients with leptomeningeal carcinomatosis without treatment is four to six weeks.[2] Outcomes from standard craniospinal radiation therapy for carcinomatous meningitis are generally poor, resulting in a median survival of only a few months; therefore, radiotherapy is surely not of primary value in providing a major survival benefit. However, in many clinical instances, it relieves symptoms, or halts rapid progression of neurologic symptoms such as cranial neuropathies. The latter constitutes the major benefit of radiotherapy and several review papers have summarized small single institutional experiences. In one of the more modern such series, Hermann, et al, evaluated the efficacy and feasibility of craniospinal irradiation with and without intrathecal chemotherapy, specifically as it pertains to symptom palliation and survival. Sixteen patients with leptomeningeal carcinomatosis (nine breast cancer, five lung cancer, one unknown primary and one renal cancer) received 36 Gy craniospinal radiotherapy (1.6-2 Gy/fraction), ten of whom also received two to eight cycles of intrathecal methotrexate at 15 mg/cycle. The overall median survival was 12 weeks; patients receiving craniospinal irradiation alone had a median survival of eight weeks, compared to 16 weeks for those patients receiving both methotrexate and craniospinal irradiation. The combined approach, although tested in only a small cohort, appeared more efficacious from a survival point-of-view. Over two-thirds of patients[9] experienced regression of their neurological symptoms either during or within days after radiotherapy was completed, outlining its palliative efficacy. Particularly impressive was the observation that seven previously non-ambulatory patients regained ambulation, six had substantial pain reduction, and three patients experienced restitution of bladder and bowel continence. All of these functional domains: ambulation, sphincter control and pain, represent critically important elements in terms of quality-of-life improvement and justify the use of craniospinal irradiation, with or without intrathecal methotrexate in selected patients with leptomeningeal carcinomatosis. However, approximately one-third of patients developed grade 3 myelosuppression; dysphagia, mucositis and nausea were relatively common. These side effects may be controlled with appropriate medications and should not necessarily preclude the use of CSI.[9]

With the increasing use of intrathecal chemotherapy, the optimal role of radiotherapy is called into question. No randomized trials have addressed this issue directly; however, one randomized study of two different chemotherapy approaches supported the use of radiotherapy. A prospective randomized trial of intrathecal methotrexate (MTX) versus MTX plus cytosine arabinoside (Ara-C) found that concurrent radiotherapy to the CNS was associated with significantly better response (73% v 35%; $P < 0.05$). Overall median survival for the whole group was eight weeks, but responders fared better than nonresponders (median survival, 18 v 7 weeks). Since radiation enhanced the response rate and responders lived longer, this trial indirectly supports the up-front use of radiotherapy with intrathecal methotrexate.[10]

3. LOCALIZED RADIATION

Because of the complicated set-up of craniospinal irradiation, the associated toxicities, and the near complete incurability of leptomeningeal cancer, most clinicians choose localized radiation instead of treating the entire craniospinal axis. Areas of high tumor burden or symptomatic regions are treated palliatively. Most often this entails whole brain irradiation and/or segmental spinal cord/cauda equina irradiation. Depending on the radiosensitivity of the tumor, radiation may be successful at relieving pain, focal weakness, sensory loss, bowel/bladder dysfunction, focal seizures, cranial nerve palsies, and cerebral spinal fluid flow abnormalities. Localized treatment ports are usually radiated with 20-40 Gy in daily fractions of 2-4 Gy. Treatment goals are based on the patient's symptoms, duration of symptoms, tumor type, and general performance status.

From 1981 through 1985, the Southwest Oncology Group (SWOG) conducted a study evaluating the natural history and the effectiveness of standard therapy in patients with leptomeningeal carcinomatosis.[11] Those patients who responded to therapy in one month exhibited a median additional survival of 5.7 months, and those who were not responders at one month exhibited a median additional survival of 1.8 months. The authors were unable to identify pre-treatment characteristics that would predict for a favorable response to therapy. These results indicate that in some patients, focal irradiation may be beneficial and aggressive treatment in some patients may be indicated, as those patients who respond to treatment have a survival benefit.[11]

Another interesting approach for localized therapy has focused on the CSF flow-impingement patterns created by the disease. Technetium-99m-DTPA flow studies within the CSF were performed in 31 patients after placement of Ommaya reservoirs. Two millicuries of Tc-99 were injected into the reservoir. Planar images of the head and entire spine were obtained after 10 and 30 minutes and after 1, 4, 6, and 24 hours. Follow-up studies were performed in 12 patients whose initial studies were abnormal or who developed complications of therapy. In 19 of the 31 patients (61%), ventricular-outlet, spinal, or convexity blocks were identified. In 11 of these 19 patients, focal radiotherapy to the site of the block restored normal flow. Survival among patients with initially normal, abnormal but correctable, and abnormal but uncorrectable CSF flow differed significantly (6.9, 13.0, and 0.7 months, respectively). The authors concluded that CSF flow blocks are common in patients with carcinomatous meningitis and may occur at the skull base, the spinal canal, and over the convexities. These flow abnormalities often can be corrected with appropriately directed radiotherapy. They also recommended that intrathecal chemotherapy should be preceded by a radionuclide flow study and be delayed if abnormal flow is documented until appropriate radiotherapy re-establishes normal flow.[12]

4. INTRATHECAL ISOTOPE THERAPY

The limitations of external beam radiotherapy, whether to the entire neuraxis, or localized, have prompted the investigation of intrathecal isotope delivery techniques which although promising, are in their infancy. In general, three approaches can be utilized: 1) direct intrathecal administration of an isotope; 2) delivery of the isotope to tumor cells using a "homing" molecule specific for cancer cells; or 3) use of isotopes tagged to large microspheres that remain localized within the CSF space. The latter approach has been tested in experimental systems using radioactive iodine 125 labeled 5-iodo-2'-deoxyuridine. This thymidine analog incorporates into the nuclei of dividing cells. The Auger electrons emitted by the I-125 bound to it are highly effective in neoplastic meningitis in rats, suggesting a potentially new therapeutic avenue for the human counterpart.[13] Other investigators are exploring radioimmunoconjugates labeled with alpha particles, such as Bismuth-212 or Astatine-211, which emit high energy radiation, but with limited tissue penetration of 100 microns or less. Preliminary in-vivo results are encouraging.[14]

The largest reported experience with radioimmunoconjugate therapy for this disease comes from Kemshead's group in the United Kingdom in which they summarized their experience from 1984 to 1993.[15] Monoclonal antibodies (MoAbs) radiolabeled with iodine 131 were administered into the CSF of 52 patients with neoplastic meningitis. The MoAbs were selected based on immunoreactivity with each patient's tumor and lack of binding to normal CNS tissue. All patients underwent full neuroimaging, which included an isotope flow study of CSF pathways. Subsequently, I 131-MoAb was administered via a ventricular access device, lumbar catheter or both. Isotope activity varied from 25 to 160 mCi. Distribution of (131)I-MAb and clearance kinetics were derived from serial scintigraphy and CSF/blood sampling. Evidence of localization to tumor was frequently observed; toxicity was minimal and easily treated. The best results were obtained in primitive neuroectodermal tumor, where 53% of evaluable cases had responses and 11% had stable disease, adults responding better than children. Three exceptional survivals were recorded; one patient leading a normal life at 10 years 11 months, one alive and normal at three years, two months, and a third surviving in good condition for eight years. The mean survival of responders was 39 months and non-responders four months. In the entire series, 50% of patients survived for at least one year. Results of treating leukemia and carcinoma suggested that re-seeding into the CSF compartment from active systemic disease accounted for early relapse in the CNS. One patient with carcinoma and no apparent systemic disease had a remarkable response and survived for four years following a single treatment.[15] In another report by the same group, a monoclonal antibody (UJ181.4) was labeled with radioactive iodine 131 which emits gamma irradiation and was administered intrathecally to a patient with neoplastic meningitis from disseminated pineoblastoma. The target antigen had first been demonstrated to be present on tumor cells by immunocytological testing of CSF. Good evidence of in vivo immunolocalization was first obtained by external gamma counting for a test dose of 131I-UJ181.4 antibody. A single relatively small therapeutic dose of 131-I (870 MBq) given by the intrathecal route, resulted in a marked clinical improvement and sustained remission for 22 months.[16]

The radiolabeled immunoconjugate approach requires intrathecal administration to overcome the limitations of poor penetration into the CSF from intravenous administration, and also to minimize the human anti-mouse antibody (HAMA) response, since most of the MoAbs are of mouse clonality. Detailed pharmacodynamic assessment of patients receiving this intracompartmental-targeted therapy demonstrates that the elimination from the ventricular CSF is biphasic with more rapid clearance occurring in the first 24 hours. From this information, the areas under the effective activity curves for ventricular CSF, blood, and subarachnoid CSF have been calculated to permit dosimetry. A marked advantage could be demonstrated for the dose delivered to tumor cells within the CSF as compared to other neural elements.[17]

In another dosimetric study, five patients with GD2-positive leptomeningeal carcinomatosis were injected with 1-2 mCi intra-Ommaya I 131-3F8, a murine IgG3 antibody specific for GD2. Serial CSF and serum samples and SPECT imaging at 4, 24, and 48 hours post-administration, were performed to determine radiation doses to the tumor and normal brain and blood prior to the administration of larger therapeutic doses. Focal I 131-3F8 uptake consistent with tumor localization was seen along the craniospinal axis in four patients. Calculated radiation dose to the CSF was 14.9-56 cGy/mCi and to blood and other organs outside the CNS less than 2 cGy/mCi. Intraventricular I 131-3F8 successfully localized to leptomeningeal disease, resulting in a favorable CSF/blood ratio.[18]

A dramatic example of neurologic improvement and long-term survival was reported by Cokgor et al.[19] A 46-year-old female presenting with progressive hearing loss, severe headaches, nausea, vomiting, and rapid decline in neurologic status was enrolled in a Phase I trial of I 131-labeled monoclonal antibody Mel-14 F(ab')(2) fragment administered intrathecally. Within a year after her treatment she recovered, having a normal neurologic exam except for residual bilateral hearing loss. As of the publication date of 2001, the patient remained neurologically normal except for a mild bilateral hearing loss more than four years after treatment and free of radiographic evidence of neoplastic meningitis.

The microsphere approach is being tested with high energy beta-emitting radioisotopes such as Yttrium-90, which have a path-length of approximately 8-10 mm. A matrix-type polymeric drug delivery system, poly lactic acid (PLA), has been designed in the form of microsphere carriers for the ionic form of 90Y. This radiopharmaceutical can be selectively delivered to a target site after incorporating 10% Fe3O4 (magnetite) which makes the magnetic microspheres responsive to an external magnetic field. These 10-40 micron diameter magnetic microspheres are biodegradable and slowly hydrolyze to lactic acid after radioactive decay. Stability studies showed that approximately 95% of added 90Y is retained within the PLA matrix after 28 days (>10 half-lives). Cytotoxicity studies with neuroblastoma cells growing in monolayer showed that the radiocytotoxicity of the microspheres could be directed magnetically to either kill or spare specific cell populations, thus making them of great interest for targeted intracavitary tumor therapy. This system is currently being optimized for use in the treatment of neoplastic meningitis.[20]

5. TREATMENT-RELATED TOXICITIES

Toxicities of radiotherapy may limit the dose that can be delivered. These toxicities range from mild and temporary to more serious and potentially permanent and debilitating. Side effects are divided into acute and delayed toxicities. Acute toxicities, which generally are temporary, include hair loss, skin reaction, sore throat, dysphagia, Eustachian tube dysfunction with "plugged ears", nausea and vomiting, and fatigue. In patients with leptomeningeal spread of their primary cancer, acute toxicities often are more concerning because the patient may not live long enough to experience long-term problems. Certain patients, however, attain longer survival and maybe at risk for delayed toxicities.

Radiation therapy may contribute to both acute and chronic bone marrow suppression, especially when large fields, such as craniospinal irradiation, are treated. Decreases in blood counts are heightened in patients who have previously received myelosuppressive chemotherapy. Because of this, more limited involved field radiation ports are used to treat the bulk of disease rather than the entire craniospinal axis. If further chemotherapy is contemplated, care should be taken to encompass the bulky disease only in order to spare bone marrow reserve.

Damage to the CNS is another serious potential toxicity of radiation treatment for leptomeningeal cancer. CNS damage is multifactorial and is dependent on total dose, dose per fraction, treatment volume and patient-related factors such as other medical co-morbidities. CNS toxicities can occur at any time, but certain problems have typical time appearances. Acute toxicities occur within the first few weeks, early-delayed toxicity from four weeks to four months, and late-delayed toxicity from four months to years after radiation.[25] Important examples include acute radiation encephalopathy, early-delayed cerebral necrosis, and late-delayed cranial nerve damage. The spinal cord also is at risk with toxicities including acute Lhermitte's sign, late-delayed radiation myelopathy, and late-delayed motor neuron syndrome. As with bone marrow toxicity, all of these complications may be potentiated with chemotherapy, particularly with intrathecal chemotherapy. These complications can confound the oncologist as they may be mistaken for disease progression.

6. CONCLUSIONS

Although carcinomatous meningitis is a relatively uncommon sequelae of malignancy, its consequences are devastating. The overall prognosis for most patients with leptomeningeal carcinomatosis is poor. The management remains controversial and categorical recommendations are difficult to make. In the absence of therapy, median survival is in the order of four to six weeks. Craniospinal irradiation may prolong this to a few months, and some studies indicate that the administration of intrathecal chemotherapy with radiation may yield slightly longer survival. Because of concerns regarding radiation side effects such as myelosuppression or mucositis, several investigators have utilized localized radiation approaches. The simplest of these is whole brain radiotherapy, which primarily targets the cranial neuropathies commonly encountered in this disease. A clinical trial reported by SWOG indicated that whole brain irradiation could be combined with chemotherapy, and the 1-month post-treatment response was highly predictive for overall survival.[11] Other more innovative localized approaches have utilized technetium ventriculography to identify sites of CSF flow occlusion which, when treated with local-field radiotherapy, frequently result in restoration of flow and relief of obstructive symptoms. Targeted radioisotope approaches are in their infancy, and a number of innovative preclinical and early clinical studies appear exciting. Regardless of the approach, radiotherapy does result in useful palliation, including return of ambulation, relief of pain and restoration of sphincter function. Not all patients with this disease fare equally poorly. Those with good performance status, limited systemic disease without fixed neurologic deficits, and with certain "sensitive" tumor types such as breast cancer, and several pediatric hematologic tumors have a better prognosis. Unfortunately, the therapeutic approaches in this disease have not been tested using rigorous clinical trial methodology, primarily because of nihilism, but also because many of these patients are often too ill to be eligible for very aggressive interventions. In an effort to stimulate randomized comparisons of various treatment approaches, Jayson, et al, summarized the problems inherent in interpreting the current literature.[26] They surmised that recommendations are difficult to make because: 1) Most series include patients with carcinomatous meningitis (CM) that has arisen from different primary malignancies which are associated with different median survival intervals. 2) There have been no prospective randomized investigations of treatment modalities in patients with CM from a particular tumor type. 3) The definition of response varies from one report to another so that some response rates refer to cytological changes in the CSF while others take clinical, cytological and biochemical parameters into account. 4) Reports include patients with and without parenchymal metastases and the natural history of CM in the two situations may differ. They further point out that the two most important endpoints for the patient, neurological improvement and overall survival, are seldom used consistently in the literature. Many reports have focused on surrogate markers of response, namely biochemical and cytological data points, but the correlation between clinical status and these parameters is poor because of differences between lumbar and ventricular CSF and disturbances of CSF flow in this disease. Multicenter, prospective, randomized trials should be strongly encouraged and conducted to address questions of most relevance to the patient, namely neurological status and overall survival.[26]

REFERENCES

1. Wasserstrom WR, Glass JP, Posner JB. Diagnosis and treatment of leptomeningeal metastases from solid tumors: experience with 90 patients. Cancer 1982; 49:759-772.

2. Grossman SA, Krabak MJ. Leptomeningeal carcinomatosis. Cancer Treat Rev 1999; 25:103-119.

3. Seeldrayers P, Hildebrand J. Treatment of neoplastic meningitis. Euro J Cancer Clin Oncol 1984; 20:449-456.

4. Iaconetta G, Lamaida E, Rossi A, Signorelli F, Manto A, Giamundo, A. Leptomeningeal carcinomatosis: review of the literature. Acta Neurologica 1009; 16:214-220.

5. Blaney SM, Poplack DG. Neoplastic meningitis: diagnosis and treatment considerations. Med Oncol 2000; 17:151-162.

6. Kagan AR. In: Perez, C.A. and Brady, L.W. (eds). Principles and Practice of Radiation Oncology, 3rd ed., Lippincott-Raven Publishers, p. 2195, 1998.

7. Das, RK. Field Matching. University of Wisconsin-Madison Radiation Physics Class. May, 2001.

8. Kun LE. In: Perez, C.A. and Brady, L.W. (eds). Principles and Practice of Radiation Oncology, 3rd ed., Lippincott-Raven Publishers, p. 2079, 1998.

9. Hermann B, Hultenschmidt B, Sautter-Bihl ML. Radiotherapy of the neuraxis for palliative treatment of leptomeningeal carcinomatosis. Strahlentherapie und Onkologie 2001; 177:195-199.

10. Hitchins RN, Bell DR, Woods RL, Levi JA. A prospective randomized trial of single-agent versus combination chemotherapy in meningeal carcinomatosis. J Clin Oncol 1987; 5:1655-1662.

11. Sause WT, Crowley J, Eyre HJ, et al. Whole brain irradiation and intrathecal methotrexate in the treatment of solid tumor leptomeningeal metastases--a Southwest Oncology Group study. J Neuro-Oncol 1988; 6:107-112, 1988.

12. Glantz MJ, Hall WA, Cole BF, et al. Diagnosis, management, and survival of patients with leptomeningeal cancer based on cerebrospinal fluid-flow status. Cancer 1995; 75:2919-2931.

13. Kassis AI, Wen PY, Van den Abbeele AD, et al. 5-[125I]iodo-2'-deoxyuridine in the radiotherapy of brain tumors in rats. J Nuclear Med 1998; 39:1148-1154.

14. Zalutsky MR, Bigner DD. Radioimmunotherapy with alpha-particle emitting radioimmunoconjugates. Acta Oncologica 1996; 35:373-379.

15. Coakham HB, Kemshead JT. Treatment of neoplastic meningitis by targeted radiation using (131)I-radiolabelled monoclonal antibodies. Results of responses and long term follow-up in 40 patients. J Neuro-Oncol 1998; 38:225-232.

16. Coakham HB, Richardson RB, Davies AG, Bourne SP, Eckert H, Kemshead JT. Neoplastic meningitis from a pineal tumour treated by antibody-guided irradiation via the intrathecal route. Br J Neurosurg 1988; 2:199-209.

17. Papanastassiou V, Pizer BL, Chandler CL, Zananiri TF, Kemshead JT, Hopkins KI. Pharmacokinetics and dose estimates following intrathecal administration of 131I-monoclonal antibodies for the treatment of central nervous system malignancies. Int J Radiat Oncol, Biol, Physics 1995; 31:541-552.

18. Kramer K, Cheung NK, Humm JL, et al. Targeted radioimmunotherapy for leptomeningeal cancer using (131)I-3F8. Med Pediat Oncol 2000; 35:716-718.

19. Cokgor I, Akabani G, Friedman HS, et al. Long term response in a patient with neoplastic meningitis secondary to melanoma treated with (131)I-radiolabeled antichondroitin proteoglycan sulfate Mel-14 F(ab')(2): a case study. Cancer 2001; 91:1809-1813.

20. Hafeli UO, Sweeney SM, Beresford BA, Sim EH, Macklis RM: Magnetically directed poly (lactic acid) 90Y-microspheres: novel agents for targeted intracavitary radiotherapy. J Biomed Materials Res 1994; 28:901-908.
21. Chamberlain MC, Kormanik PR. Carcinomatous meningitis secondary to breast cancer: predictors of response to combined modality therapy. J Neuro-Oncol 1997; 35:55-64.
22. Lampl Y, Paniri Y, Eshel Y, Sarova-Pinchas I. Alkaline phosphatase level in CSF in various brain tumors and pulmonary carcinomatous meningitis. J Neuro-Oncol 1990; 9:35-40.
23. Chamberlain MC. Pediatric leptomeningeal metastases: outcome following combined therapy. J Child Neurol 1997; 12:53-59.
24. Jennings MT, Slatkin N, D'Angelo M, et al. Neoplastic meningitis as the presentation of occult primitive neuroectodermal tumors. J Child Neurol 1993; 8:306-312.
25. Hanssens PEJ, Lagerwaard FJ, Levendag PC. Principles of radiotherapy of neoplastic meningosis. J Neuro-Oncol 1998; 38:145-150.
26. Jayson GC, Howell A. Carcinomatous meningitis in solid tumours. Ann Oncol 1996; 7:773-786.

Chapter 10

ANIMAL MODELS OF LEPTOMENINGEAL CANCER

Ali Raja, M.D. and Herbert H. Engelhard, M.D., Ph.D.
University of Illinois at Chicago, Chicago, IL 60612

Abstract: Animal models are a critical tool for our understanding of pathogenic mechanisms and the development of therapeutic strategies. Since the 1970's, numerous syngeneic and allogeneic rodent models of leptomeningeal cancer have been developed; in this chapter, we present representative models and discuss their clinical and translational implications.

Key words: Syngeneic, allogeneic, xenogenic; animal models; leptomeningeal cancer; translational research

1. INTRODUCTION

Since its initial description in a landmark paper by Eberth[1] in 1870, significant advancements in the understanding and treatment of leptomeningeal cancer (LC) have been made through the use of experimental animal models. These models have provided a useful means for *in vivo* evaluation of various potential chemotherapeutic agents and other anti-neoplastic treatment modalities including intrathecal immunotherapy and gene therapy.

In scientific research, modeling provides a practical approach for investigating the normal and abnormal function of living organisms.[2] By constructing a model, the problem being studied is simulated as accurately as possible. Using animal models, experiments can be performed that are not feasible with living human subjects or patients. Unfortunately, despite decades of research in this field, there are few animal models that accurately parallel the clinical condition in humans.[3]

Reports of experimental models for LC were first published in the mid-1970's.[4] Murine animal models have traditionally been used for testing the chemosensitivity of cancer cells. The models for LC in the literature can be divided into two categories: 1) syngeneic, and 2) allogeneic/xenogeneic. In *syngeneic* models, animal tumor cell lines are implanted into a genetically identical host. In *allogeneic* models, genetically dissimilar cells are implanted into an immunocompromised host. If species lines are crossed, the model is actually *xenogeneic*. The earlier animal models of LC were typically syngeneic using mice, rats, rabbit or guinea pigs. Recently, allogeneic and xenogeneic models using nude mice and nude rats have also been developed. The advantage of using the latter type of models is that human tumor cell lines can be used and tested. Many of the syngeneic and xenogeneic models for LC are listed according to the type of tumor cell line in Tables 1 and 2, respectively.

One potential problem in treating malignant tumors of the central nervous system (CNS) and/or the meninges is inadequate drug delivery across the blood-brain barrier (BBB).[5-8] Systemically administered hydrophilic (and even lipid soluble) drugs usually penetrate the CNS parenchyma for short distances[9] and thus fail to reach tumor cells in sufficient concentrations. Intrathecal injection of drugs directly into the cerebrospinal fluid (CSF) has been used to circumvent this problem with the rationale that high concentrations of the drug may be achieved in the vicinity of tumor located on the meninges. Most animal models involve the use of the intrathecal drug delivery method for this purpose. Animals are usually prepared by direct inoculation of tumor cells into brain parenchyma or by intracisternal inoculation.

Table 1. Syngeneic Animal Models of Leptomeningeal Cancer

Tumor Type	Cell Line	Animal	Experiment	Reference
Glioma	C6 glioma	Wistar rat	ACNU, BCNU, VM26	Yoshida,1984 [10]
			Model	Yoshida,1986 [11]
			it neocarzinostatin	Yoshida,1987 [12]
			it ACNU	Yoshida ,1992 [13]
			it IL-2	Herrlinger,1996 [14]
	9L glioma	Fischer rat	ACNU, BCNU, VM26	Yoshida,1984 [10]
			Model	Yoshida,1986 [11]
			it ACNU	Yoshida,1992 [13]
			Model	Kooistra,1986 [15]
			Model	Rewers,1990 [16]
			it gene therapy (retroviral vector-mediated HS-TK gene transfer)	Ram,1994 [17]
			it gene therapy (herpes simplex I-thymidine kinase)	Kramm,1996 [18]
			herpes simplex I- thymidine kinase/ganciclovir paradigm	Kramm,1996 [19]
			it gene therapy (adenovirus)	Vincent,1996 [20]
			it MGH-1 viral vector-mediated gene therapy	Kramm,1997 [21]
			it ^{125}IudR	Sahu,1997 [22]
Carcinoma	W256 ca	Walker rat	Model	Ushio,1977 [4]
			it/iv cyclophosphamide, CCNU, methyl-CCNU, methotrexate, cytarabine	Ushio,1977 [23]
			iv cyclophosphamide, ACNU	Ushio,1981 [24]
			iv cyclophosphamide, bleomycin	Shimizu,1980 [25]
			Model	Kooistra,1986 [15]
			it bleomycin, cytarabine, dacarbazine, doxorubicin, 5-fluorouracil, methotrexate, mitomycin C, thiotepa, BCNU	Kooistra,1989 [26]
			iv diaziquone, methotrexate	
			effects of LC on brain parenchyma	Jamshidi,1987 [27]
			growth kinetics of LC	Izumoto,1988 [28]
			model/ brain glucose metabolism	Hiesiger,1989 [29]
			it ACNU	Huang,1997 [30]
			estimating proliferating activity in LC	Huang,1997 [31]
			it gene therapy (W256 cells transfected *in vitro*)	Vrionis,1996 [32]
	MAT BIII rmc	Fischer rat	model/immune response	Sagar,1995 [33]
	VX2	NZW rb	Model	Miree,1972 [34]
			model/relationship of number of tumor cells and survival	Miree, 1973 [35]
			model/ MRI study	Frank,1988 [36]
			it 4-HC	Phillips,1992 [37]

Table 1. (Continued)

Abbreviations: it, intrathecal; ca, carcinoma; iv, intravenous; mo, mouse; gp, guinea pig; rmc, rat mammary carcinoma, rb, rabbit; sc, subcutaneous.

Tumor Type	Cell line	Animal	Experiment	Reference
Melanoma	B16-B14b	Mo	Model	Miner,1982 [38]
	B16-F10	Mo	iv doxorubicin/ blood-brain barrier function	Seigal,1987 [39]
Leukemia	L1210	Mo	Model/sc cyclophosphamide	Thomas,1962;1964 [40, 41]
			sc antifolate/ ip immunization with irradiated L1210 cells	Chirigos,1964 [42]
			sc methotrexate, BCNU, cytoxan	Chirigos,1966 [43]
	LL	Mo	ip amphotericin B, BCNU	Lynch,1975 [44]
	L5222 AML	Mo	ip/sc BCNU, cyclophosphamide	Fiebig,1976 [45]
	T cell	Mo	Model	Varakis,1982 [46]
	DBLA6	Rat	iv daunomycin/ blood-brain barrier function	Suzuki,1983 [47]
	L4414 ALL	Rat	Model	Hoogerbrugge,1985 [48]
	BNML AML	Rat	Model	Hoogerbrugge,1985 [48]
	L2C	Gp	immunotoxin	Urch,1991 [49]
			it immunotoxin	Zovickian,1988 [50]
			Model	Perk,1974 [51]
Lymphoma	NHL	Mo	Model	Peterson,1980 [52]
			Model	Kupper,1987 [53]
	S49	Mo	it vaccination with live immunogeneic variants of S49 cells	Siegal,1986 [54]

Table 2. Xenogeneic Animal Models of Leptomeningeal Cancer

Tumor	Cell Line	Animal	Experiment	Reference
Glioma	hu cell lines	nu mo	model	Yoshida,1986 [55]
	hu ONS-6,12,16	nu mo	model	Miyao,1986 [56]
	hu ONS-12	nu mo	ip/it IFN-β	Miyao,1987 [57]
	hu U87	nu mo	ip BCNU/ it methotrexate	Abernathey,1988 [58]
			it monoclonal antibodies/ MRI	Yamashita,1993 [59]
	hu D54	nu rat	it mafosfamide/ functional tests	Fuchs,1990 [60]
	D-54 MG	nu rat	it melphalan	Friedman,1994 [61]
	hu SNB19	nu rat	model	Bergman,1997 [62]
	hu U87	nu rat	model	Bergman,1997 [62]
Breast Cancer	hu SKBR3	nu rat	model	Bergman,1997 [62]
Neuroblastoma	hu IMR-32	nu rat	model	Bergman,1997 [62]
	hu NMB7	nu rat	model	Bergman,1997 [62]
Medulloblastoma	hu ONS-76	nu mo	model/ MHC class I expression	Yamada,1991 [63]
	hu MHH-MED-1	nu rat	model/ MRI	Schabet,1997 [64]
	hu DAOY	nu rat	model	Janczewski,1998 [3]
			adeno-associated virus vector transduction	Rosenfeld,1997 [65]
			model	Bergman,1997 [62]
	hu D283	nu rat	model	Bergman,1997 [62]
Carcinoma	hu 146 SCLC	nu rat	it immunotoxin	Myklebust,1994 [11]
	hu DMS-273 SCLC	nu rat	model	Myklebust,1994 [67]
	hu A431	nu rat	it immunotoxin	Pastan,1995 [68]
	hu MDA-MB 231 br ca	nu rat	model	Janczewski,1998 [3]
	hu SKBR3	nu rat	model	Bergman,1997 [62]
	hu MCF7	nu rat	model	Bergman,1997 [62]

Table 2. (Continued)

Tumor	Cell Line	Animal	Experiment	Reference
Melanoma	mo B16-F10	nu rat	Model	Schabet,1987 [69]
			it ACNU	Schabet,1992 [70]
			it methotrexate, IFN-γ, TNF-α	Schabet,1994 [71]
			model/ MRI	Martos,1992 [72]
	hu Mel-1	nu rat	model	Bergman,1997 [62]
	hu Mel-28	nu rat	model	Bergman,1997 [62]
	hu SK-MEL-28	nu rat	model	Schabet,1987 [69]
	hu Me Wo	nu rat	model	Schabet,1994 [73]
	hu LOX	nu rat	model	Myklebust,1994 [67]
			it immunotoxin	Hall,1994 [74]
	hu B16F-10	nu mo	model	Reijneveld,1999 [75]
Sarcoma	hu TE-671	nu rat	it mafosfamide	Fuchs,1990 [60]
	hu TE-671	nu rat	it melphalan	Friedman,1994 [61]
	hu TE-671	nu rat	it radioimmuno-conjugate	Zalutsky,1994 [76]
Leukemia	DBLA-6	nu rat	model/ACNU, CCNU, procarbazine	Kobayashi,1985 [77]
	hu PF382	nu mo	model	Cavallo,1992 [78]
	hu CEM	nu rat	it immunotoxin	Herrlinger,1996 [79]
Lymphoma	hu Raji bl	nu rat	P-4055 & cytarabine	Breistøl,1999 [80]
	hu NHL	nu mo	model	Epstein,1976 [81]
	hu ST-4	nu mo	model	Cavallo,1992 [78]

Abbreviations: it, intrathecal; nu, nude; mo, mouse; gp, guinea pig; hu, human; br ca, breast carcinoma; osteo sar, osteogenic sarcoma; bl, Burkitt's lymphoma.

Most of the animal models have been specifically developed for the purpose of evaluating a certain treatment modality against a particular form of leptomeningeal cancer. However, some of the studies simply analyzed the model itself. For example, Yamada et al[63] developed an experimental model of meningeal dissemination by intracisternal inoculation of human medulloblastoma (ONS-76) cells into nude mice. They used immunohistochemical studies to show that ONS-76 cells in the subarachnoid space expressed major histocompatibility (MHC) class I antigens until 20 days after inoculation. After 30 days, expression of MHC class I antigens decreased and the tumor cells began to proliferate rapidly. Similarly, Yoshida and colleagues[82,11] developed experimental models of LC by intracisternal inoculation of rat C6 and 9L glioma cells into Wistar and Fischer rats, respectively. They studied the clinico-pathological features in both models and found them to be similar to those seen with gliomas in humans. In another paper, Kooistra et al[15] reported development of 9L gliosarcoma and Walker 256 carcinosarcoma models in rats and described the tumor cell dose response, functional and behavioral changes, and the histology in each model. Some other models were developed specifically for studying one or the other aspect of the disease. For example, Hiesiger et al developed a LC model using Walker 256 tumor cells in rats to study the effect of the tumor on cerebral glucose utilization (LCGU). They observed that the tumor resulted in selective regional depression of LCGU that occurred both in structures underlying the tumor and those anatomically remote, but in certain cases, functionally related to structures subjacent to the tumor. Similarly, Siegal et al[39] developed a B_{16} melanoma model in C57BL mice for studying the alteration of blood-brain-CSF barrier using Evans blue and Horseradish peroxidase tracers. Brain concentrations of Adriamycin following an intravenous dose were also studied and a significant increase in its content in the whole brain was observed as compared with the tumor free controls ($P < 0.05$). The study concluded that although an alteration in the barrier allows extravasation of the tracer, a high-dose regimen is required to achieve a significant increase in a water-soluble drug penetration through the disrupted barrier. Most other models in the literature either analyze one or more aspects (e.g. pharmacokinetics and toxicity) of a potential anti-neoplastic treatment modality or look at the efficacy of a treatment option against a specific tumor type.

Different studies use different cell lines to mimic LC. Since leptomeningeal dissemination occurs in 5-15% of patients with malignant gliomas and with similar frequency in patients with solid tumors like breast cancer, lung cancer, and malignant melanoma,[83,84] most researchers have used tumor cells from one of these tumors in their models. Others have used lymphoma cells due to the high rate of LC seen in acute lymphoblastic leukemia (ALL) patients.[82,85]

The following are some examples of these experimental models for LC that were developed for testing chemotherapeutic, immunotherapeutic or gene therapy agents.

2. MODELS TESTING CHEMOTHERAPEUTIC AGENTS

Almost all of the earlier experiments and many of the newer ones tested one or another potential chemotherapeutic agent. Toxicity to normal CNS tissue is an important consideration for many of these agents. Through animal testing, the safety of these agents can be determined before the development of human trials. Brain tumor models with human tumor cell lines in nude rats and mice have led to identification of human chemotherapies. Results from representative studies are summarized below.

2.1 Nude rat model using B16-F10 melanoma cells for evaluating effects of intrathecal ((1-4-amino-2-metyl-5-pyrimidinyl)methyl-3-(2-chloroethyl)-3-nitrosourea hydrochloride) or ACNU

In a study by Schabet et al,[70] a single or repeated non-toxic dose of 1 mg/kg of ACNU was injected into the cisterna magna of rats inoculated with the tumor. Median symptom-free survival was 16 days (range, 14-27) for controls (n = 9) and 18 days (range, 17-23) for rats treated with ACNU on day 4 (n = 9). Animals treated both on day 2 and 8 (n = 8) developed symptoms on day 21 (range, 13-35). Based on these results along with the pharmacokinetic data on the drug, the study concluded that although bolus injection of ACNU is locally effective, it is not sufficient for treating widespread leptomeningeal metastases.

2.2 Rat model of Walker 256 carcinosarcoma cells for intrathecal ACNU

Huang and Howng[30] studied the therapeutic efficacy and cell kinetics of intrathecal ACNU in rats using a meningeal carcinomatosis model induced by intracisternal inoculation of Walker 256 carcinosarcoma cells. The median survival time of the rats treated with intrathecal ACNU (1.5 mg/kg on day 5 after tumor inoculation) was significantly increased by 145% in comparison with the untreated rats. The cell kinetics were studied immunohistochemically using indirect immunoperoxidase method with bromodeoxyuridine (BrdU) and anti-BrdU monoclonal antibody (Becton-Dickinson). Before and 12, 24, 48, 96 or 144 hours after treatment with ACNU, the rats received intravenous BrdU (200 mg/kg) injection. Thirty minutes later, the rats were sacrificed and the brains removed. Sections of the brain were stained with anti-BrdU monoclonal antibody. A labeling index (LI) (the percentage of tumor cells in the synthetic phase) was obtained by counting the immunoreactive cells under the microscope. The index was 34% in the group that was stained before treatment and dropped to below 20% in the groups stained 12 to 48 hours post-treatment. However, it increased to about 36% on the fourth post-treatment day. The investigators concluded that a greater anti-neoplastic effect of intrathecal ACNU against meningeal carcinomatosis might be expected in the earlier stage of intrathecal administration.

The same group (Huang et al[31]) reported the immunohistochemical results from a study that used a similar model but without any treatment groups. The LI was as low as10.8% to 16.9% in the first days after tumor inoculation and increased to 24.0% to 40.1% after 4-6 days. The LI reached a plateau seven to nine days post-inoculation at 40.7% to 48.2%. At day ten when necrosis appeared in the tumor, BrdU-positive cells declined and LI fell between 29.1% and 35.0%.

2.3 Rat C6 glioma model for testing intrathecal ACNU chemotherapy

In the study by Yoshida et al,[13] the median survival time of the rats treated with a single dose of intrathecal ACNU (1 mg/kg) on day one or three after tumor inoculation was significantly prolonged by 35.7% to 42.9 or 25.55 to 28.6%, respectively, as compared with control animals. Rats treated after 5 days with intrathecal (1 mg/kg) or intravenous (15 mg/kg) drug administration, however, did not show prolonged survival times. The authors concluded that low-dose ACNU treatment might be effective if given in the early stages of the disease.

2.4 Testing intrathecal 5-[125I]iodo-2'-deoxyuridine in rats with LC from 9L rat gliosarcoma cells

In this study by Sahu et al[22], intrathecal 5-[125I]iodo-2'-deoxyuridine (125IUdR) was administered, three days after implantation of 9L rat gliosarcoma cells, as a single injection, five daily injections or as a continuous 5-day infusion. Control groups received physiologic saline. All groups were monitored for the onset of paralysis. For biodistribution studies, rats received a bolus injection of 125IudR five days after tumor cell implantation and were killed 1, 8, 24 and 48 hours later. In the treatment group, the median time to paralysis was significantly prolonged ($p \leq 0.005$) to 11.2±0.1, 12.3±0.1 and 15.2±0.4 days for the single-dose, five daily injections and continuous infusion groups, respectively. The authors concluded that a selective anti-tumor effect could be achieved in treating leptomeningeal metastases with this drug.

2.5 Testing anti-tumor activity of P-4055 compared to Cytarabine in nude rats and mice

Breistøl et al[80] studied the anti-neoplastic efficacy of P-4055 (elaidic acid-cytarabine) in several *in vivo* models using human cancer cell lines. Control animals were treated either with cytarabine or a saline solution. In a Raji

Burkitt's lymphoma LC model in nude rats, the control (cytarabine and saline treated) animals (five in each group) had a mean survival time of 13.2 days as compared to the P-4055 treated rats which had three to five times greater survival times. In the same paper, a systemic Raji leukemia cell model in nude mice showed that eight of the ten P-4055-treated animals survived more than 80 days, as compared with the cytarabine-treated animals with a mean survival time of 34.2 days. The authors also studied the efficacy of P-4055 against different solid tumor cell lines implanted subcutaneously. They concluded that based on these results, clinical trials for P-4055 were indicated.

2.6 Studying efficacy of intrathecal (NCS) in a C6 glioma cell rat leptomeningeal cancer model

In this study by Yoshida et al,[12] intrathecal Neocarzinostatin (NCS) at a dose of 1 μg/kg was administered one day after tumor inoculation. The survival time was significantly prolonged by the treatment and improved with an increase in drug dosage. The survival times decreased when the rats were treated after three days of tumor inoculation and no effect was observed when it was given after five days (even at a dose of 100 μg/kg). The authors concluded that low dose chemotherapy with NCS would be more effective if given in the early stages of leptomeningeal cancer.

2.7 Nude rat model with D-54 human glioma cells or TE-671 human rhabdomyosarcoma cells for testing 4-HC activity against leptomeningeal cancer

Fuchs et al[60] reported on the development of an animal model of LC and activity of intrathecal 4-HC against human rhabdomyosarcoma cell line TE-671 and the human glioma cell line D-54 MG. The injection of 5×10^5 TE-671 or D-54 MG cells in the subarachnoid space of athymic rats resulted in growth of LC from the base of the brain to the cauda equina. Daily weights and neurological examinations were performed and revealed progressive neurological deficits and weight loss. Deaths occurred between days 21 and 27 for TE-671 and days 14 and 26 for d-54 MG, respectively. 4-HC toxicity in non-tumor-bearing rats was assessed at dose levels of 2.0, 10.0, 15.0, and 20.0 mM, with clinical and histological evidence of neurotoxicity observed at the two highest dose levels. Intrathecal treatment with 4-HC on day eight after injection of TE-671 resulted in an increase in median survival of 20% ($P = 0.04$) at 1.0 mM 4-HC and 41% ($P < 0.001$), respectively at 2.5 mM 4-HC. Intrathecal treatment with 4-HC (2.5 mM) on day five following injection of D-54 MG resulted in an increase in median survival of 23% ($P = 0.009$). The study concluded that 4-HC was effective against these cell lines and lacked toxicity at therapeutic levels in the normal athymic rats.

2.8 Nude rat model with D-54 human glioma cells or TE-671 human rhabdomyosarcoma cells for testing intrathecal Melphalan therapy

In a study by Friedman et al[61], melphalan was administered on days eight or five depending on the tumor cell line and dose. Multiple dose toxicity studies using a 0.25, 0.5, 0.75, 1.0, 1.5, or 2.0 mM solution revealed clinical and histological evidence of dose-dependent toxicity at all dosages. Treatment of TE-671 with a single dose of 2.0 mM intrathecal melphalan produced an increase in median survival of 442% as compared to the saline controls ($P<0.003$). Comparison of the multiple, low-dose regimen with single, high dose regimen revealed a greater increase in survival times for the former. This effect was more pronounced in TE-671 inoculated rats. The authors concluded that intrathecal melphalan may be an important addition to the drugs used for the treatment of this disease.

3. MODEL TESTING IMMUNOTHERAPEUTIC AGENTS

Contemporary immunotoxins are a group of cell-type specific cytotoxic agents that are made up of a monoclonal antibody linked to a protein toxin. The current immunotherapeutic approaches for the treatment of LC include the intrathecal administration of:

1. Immunomodulating cytokines such as interleukin-2 (IL-2) and interferon-α (IFN-α).
2. Immune effector cells such as lymphokine-activated killer cells (LAK cells).

   Both of these are referred to as “active” immunotherapeutic approaches as opposed to intrathecal application of antibodies, which is termed “passive” immunotherapy. Results from rodent models testing IL-2 have not been very encouraging.[14,86] For example, in a Wistar rat model with C6 glioma cells, Herrlinger et al[14] found that intrathecal application of high-dose IL-2 elicited only a slight immune reaction within the leptomeninges and did not inhibit leptomeningeal tumor growth or prolong symptom-free survival in the animals.

3.1 Efficacy of intrathecal immunotoxin therapy in a L_2C tumor cell model in guinea pig

Zovickian et al[87] inoculated tumor cells percutaneously into the cisterna magna of the test animals. Control animals developed disseminated leptomeningeal and intraventricular leukemia and death. For treated animals, intracisternal tumor inoculation was followed by intracisternal injection of 2 μg of an anti-idiotype monoclonal antibody (M6)-intact ricin immunotoxin after 24 hours. This produced prolonged survival ($P < 0.005$) with a tumor load of 10^5 L_2C cells (10,000 times the lethal dose). The immunotoxin produced no detectable toxicity. The observed extension of survival times with the immunotherapy corresponds to a median 2- to 3-log (99% to 99.9%) and possibly a 5-log (99.999%) in some animals or greater kill of tumor cells. The study concluded that the results supported a possible role for immunotoxins in the treatment of compartmentalized CNS disorders such as those involving the intrathecal space.

3.2 Wistar rat model with C6 glioma cells for studying the efficacy of IL-2 against leptomeningeal cancer

Herrlinger et al[14] evaluated the efficacy of intrathecal treatment of LC with IL-2 in a Wistar rat model. The animals were intracisternally inoculated with 10^7 C6 glioma cells. Twelve animals were subsequently treated with intracisternal injection of 10^5 IU IL-2 or a control medium on the day of injection and days 2 and 5 after tumor cell inoculation. Both IL-2-treated and sham-treated animals developed LC with a symptom-free survival of seven to nine days. No significant difference was found between the two groups regarding time to onset of symptoms and pattern of tumor growth. Infiltration of the tumor tissue with ED-1+ monocytes and macrophages, and CD8+ lymphocytes, however, was slightly increased in animals treated with IL-2. In another set of experiments, four non-tumor bearing rats were intracisternally injected with a single dose of 10^5 IU IL-2. These animals also showed slightly enhanced leptomeningeal infiltration with CD8+ lymphocytes compared to controls. Prior to the *in vivo* experiments, the anti-proliferative effects of IL-2, murine IFN-γ, and TNF-α were also tested in a colony forming assay (IFN-γ and TNF-α are cytokines induced by IL-2). Only IFN-γ caused a dose-dependent inhibition of colony formation. The authors concluded that intrathecal application of high-dose IL-2, while eliciting a slight immune reaction within the leptomeninges, did not inhibit LC growth or prolong symptom-free survival in the animals.

3.3 Nude rat model using H-146 small cell lung cancer cells for studying targeted immunotoxin therapy

In their study, Myklebust el al[66] injected tumor cells directly into the CSF in the cisterna magna. Small, superficial leptomeningeal lesions developed with symptoms of CNS involvement after a mean latency of 20 days. They used the model to study the efficacy of MOC-31-PE immunotoxin against this tumor by instilling a single bolus dose of 1.5 micrograms into the cisterna magna. The immunotoxin was shown to increase symptom-free latency by 35-46%. Delayed or repeated treatment was less effective than day one administration, whereas the addition of 10% glycerol to the solution increased the symptom-free period to 72%. It was concluded that the results support the development of the use of this immunotoxin for treatment of patients with LC resulting from small cell lung cancer.

3.4 Acute lymphoblastic leukemia (ALL) model of LC in guinea pigs for investigating effects of intrathecal immunotoxin

In these experiments by Urch et al,[49] direct inoculation of L_2C lymphoma cells into the cisterna magna gave rise to a leptomeningeal pattern of growth similar to humans. They used an immunotoxin that consisted of an anti-idiotypic antibody disulphide-bonded to the ribosome-inactivating protein saporin. The animals received the immunotoxin into the cisterna magna one day after inoculation of L_2C cell. All animals treated with 0.5 or 5 μg of immunotoxin survived and remained tumor-free for more than 100 days after treatment. The control animals given cyclophosphamide alone or an irrelevant immunotoxin had a mean survival time of 28 days. The authors concluded that intrathecal immunotoxins offer an alternative, highly specific form of treatment for this disease.

3.5 Nude rat model using CEM T-cell lymphoma for testing intrathecal anti-CD7 ricin toxin A chain immunotoxin (DA7)

Herrlinger et al[88] treated eight animals with cisternal inoculation of 10 μg DA7 in 50 μl of phosphate buffered saline (PBS) or sham-treated with 50 μl of PBS, one and four days after cisternal inoculation of 10^6 CEM cells. Three DA7-treated animals were free of tumor; two of these were asymptomatic long-term survivors (>90 days) and the third tumor-free animal died suddenly on day 51 with histological viral myocarditis. Median symptom-free survival was 51 days (range, 29-90+ days) in DA7 treated animals and 34 days (range, 29-87 days) in sham-treated animals. No signs of neurotoxicity or systemic toxicity were found on histology. However, DA7-treated animals showed a tendency to a slower weight gain on days 6 to 28 after tumor cell inoculation. The study concluded that anti-tumor effect of DA7 needed further evaluation, especially in the early stages of LC from T-cell lymphoma.

4. MODELS TESTING GENE THERAPY

Animal models of leptomeningeal gliomatosis for studying gene therapeutic treatment approaches have appeared in the literature relatively recently. Most of the studies involve development of animal models to test the possibility of delivering gene vectors to the tumor cells. Selected studies are summarized below.

4.1 Herpes vector mediated delivery of marker genes to disseminated central nervous system tumors

Kramm et al[18] investigated the ability of a recombinant herpes simplex virus type 1 (HSV) vector, hrR3, for delivering genes into multiple brain tumor foci in adult rats. The model was developed by injecting 9L gliosarcoma cells into the right frontal lobe and in the CSF by injection through the cisterna magna. The HSV vector was inoculated intrathecally five days later. Two days after the injection of the vector, immunohistochemical staining for HSV thymidine kinase (*HSV-tk*) was performed. This revealed expression in the frontal tumors as well as in leptomeningeal tumor foci along the entire neuraxis. *HSV-tk* immunopositive cells were most frequent in small tumors contacting the CSF pathways. Frontal lobe tumors showed the highest density of *HSV-tk* immunopositive cells around their periphery with little expression in central parts. Some periventricular neurons temporarily showed immunolabeling. The number of immunopositive tumor cells markedly decreased five days after injection of the HSV vector. In all animals, some toxicity was observed in the first two to four days after vector injection in the form of extensive leptomeningeal inflammation. The authors concluded that intrathecal injection of HSV vector could mediate widespread transfer of the *HSV-tk* gene into tumors disseminated throughout the brain and CSF pathways offering a promising approach in conjunction with development of less toxic vectors. In another paper, Kramm et al[19] reported similar experiments but added systemic ganciclovir (GCV) treatment two days after vector application which continued for 14 days. Tumor-free, long-term survival was achieved in 90% of the animals treated subsequently with GCV; in 30% of those treated only with the vector and in 10% of the untreated animals. Vector-related mortality of 20% was observed in the group that did not receive subsequent GCV therapy. No mortality was seen in GCV-treated animals. Apparently, GCV was able to control HSV-related toxicity. The authors concluded that intrathecal application of HSV vectors combined with GCV treatment could be an effective approach for treating disseminated brain tumors.

In another study by Vrionis et al,[89] cells expressing *HSV-tk* were used for treating LC in Walker 256 rats. When 2×10^5 Walker cells were intrathecally injected, the median survival time was 15 days. But when *HSV-tk*-modified Walker cells were implanted and treated with ganciclovir, 80% of the rats survived for 120 days or more. The rest of the 20% died from tumor growth between 37 to 44 days after implantation. Walker TK-positive cells were better than murine fibroblast *HSV-tk* virus-producer cells in improving survival of animals with Walker tumors at low (1:1) but not at high (10:1) effector to target cell ratios. Based on these and other results, the authors concluded that Walker TK-positive cells are at least as effective as murine virus-producer cells and might be useful for the treatment of meningeal neoplasia.

Ram et al[17] implanted Fisher rats with tumor cells followed by injection of *HSV-tk* vector-producer cells in the subarachnoid space on the same day. After seven days, ganciclovir was injected intraperitoneally or intrathecally daily for 14 consecutive days. To evaluate possible enhancement of tumor eradication by the ability of helper virus to package the vector in the cells, additional rats received thymidine kinase vector-producer cells that had previously been co-infected with a replication-competent retrovirus (4070A). In all groups, control rats received intraperitoneal or intrathecal saline injections. Rats that received ganciclovir intraperitoneally after the injection of thymidine kinase vector-producer cells had significant prolongation of survival. Injection of producer cells co-infected with the 4070A retrovirus did not improve anti-tumor efficacy. Intrathecal administration of ganciclovir did not extend survival. The authors concluded that gene therapy using the thymidine kinase/ganciclovir approach had a potential application for treating leptomeningeal cancer.

4.2 9L rat brain tumor cell LC model in Fisher rats for studying a combined treatment approach with gene transduction and ganciclovir

Vincent et al[20] constructed recombinant adenoviral vectors to study their feasibility and efficacy in the palliative treatment of patients with leptomeningeal metastases. 9L brain tumor cells were injected into the CSF of Fischer rats via the cisterna magna. Three days after tumor cell injection, recombinant adenovirus containing the *lacZ* reporter gene was injected via the same route. Six days after tumor cell injection, expression of the reporter gene was detected in the tumor cells along the neuraxis. Subsequently, the experiments were repeated with tumor cell injection with *HSV-tk* three days after injection of tumor cells. Intraperitoneal GCV therapy was started the next day and continued for 10 days. Rats that developed neurological symptoms were immediately killed. The symptom-free latency of every rat was then determined. The results showed that the rats treated with *HSV-tk* and subsequent GCV had significantly longer ($P < 0.01$) symptom-free latency than the control groups. The study concluded that this approach is feasible and efficacious in a rat model and should be used in the palliative treatment of patients with leptomeningeal cancer.

4.3 Adeno-associated virus-mediated transduction in nude rat model of leptomeningeal disease with Medulloblastoma cells

Rosenfeld et al[65] used the adeno-associated virus (AAV) for transducing foreign genes into LC model using medulloblastoma cells in nude rats. This experiment was meant to be a pilot study for demonstrating that AAV vectors can be used to transfer and express foreign genes in established leptomeningeal tumors. After vector carrying the bacterial lacZ gene was injected in the ventricles, β-galactosidase-positive cells were found in the implanted tumor cells as well as in the ependymal and subependymal layers. There was no evidence of the vector in the normal brain tissue and no evidence of virally-mediated toxicity in the animals. The authors concluded that AAV vectors may be used to transfer and express foreign genes in cases of leptomeningeal cancer.

4.4 Mouse model using B16F-10 Murine melanoma cells for testing repeated intrathecal drug delivery

A paper by Reijneveld et al[75] described their model in which B16F-10 murine melanoma cells were injected intracisternally in mice producing histological characteristics comparable with human leptomeningeal metastases in humans. Recombinant adenoviral vector containing the LacZ gene was then injected intracisternally. Transfected cells were found in ependymal and subependymal cells throughout the brain but not in the parenchymal cells. The study also demonstrated the presence of continued gene expression for at least a month in immunodeficient mice without any indication of toxicity or decrease in intensity.

5. LIMITATIONS OF ANIMAL MODELS

Like all other research tools, animal models for leptomeningeal cancer have certain limitations. At best, an animal model is an approximation of not only the disease process but also the treatment method being tested as it would take place in the patients. Although these experiments pave the road towards further testing and patient trials, the results of effectiveness and toxicity may be very different from those that will actually occur in the human subjects. The debate on whether animal testing is ethical or not continues.

6. CONCLUSIONS

Animal models for LC have served a two-fold purpose. First, they have been used to determine the safety, optimal dosages and efficiency for anti-neoplastic drugs[10,24-26,39,58,61,70] and other treatment modalities.[66,57,59,68,74,79] Second, they have helped improve the understanding of the mechanisms of this disease. Results from animal studies have been applied to the clinical situation with reasonable success.[92] As the ideal treatment for malignant neoplasia involving the leptomeninges continues to elude researchers, the interest in the field of leptomeningeal models continues to grow. Newer models and innovative approaches for treatment are being developed. It is hoped that with further research using these models, a cure for this devastating complication of cancer will one day become a reality.

ACKNOWLEDGEMENTS

The authors would like to acknowledge Mariam A. Raja, B.A. for her invaluable assistance in preparing the manuscript and tables.

REFERENCES

1. Eberth CJ. Zur entwickelung des epithelioms (cholesteatoms) der pia und der lunge. Arch Pathol Anat Physiol Klin Med 1870; 49:51-63.
2. Malmivuo, Plonsey, *Bioelectromagnetism*. New York: Oxford University Press, 1995.
3. Janczewski KH, Chalk CL, Pyles RB, Parysek LM, Unger LW, Warnick RE. A simple, reproducible technique for establishing leptomeningeal tumors in nude rats. J Neurosci Methods 1998; 85:45-9.
4. Ushio Y, Chernik NL, Posner JB, Shapiro WR. Meningeal carcinomatosis: Development of an experimental model. J Neuropathol Exp Neurol 1977; 36:228-44.
5. Wilson CB, Levin VA, Sheline GC. "Management of CNS tumors in the adult patient." In *Principles of Cancer Treatment,* SK Carter, E Glatstein, RB Livingston, eds. New York, NY: McGraw-Hill, 1982.
6. Levin VA. A pharmacologic basis for tumor chemotherapy. Semin Onco 1975; 2:57-67.
7. Engelhard, Groothuis. "The blood-brain barrier: Structure, function and response to neoplasia." In *The Gliomas*, M. Berger and C. Wilson, eds. Philadelphia, PA: W.B. Saunders Co, 1998.
8. Engelhard. "Brain tumors and the blood-brain barrier." In *Neuro-Oncology: The Essentials*, M. Bernstien, M. Berger, eds. New York, NY: Thieme, 2000.
9. Levin VA, Landahl HD, Patlak CS. Drug delivery to CNS tumors. Cancer Treat Rep 1981; 65:19-25.

10. Yoshida T, Shimizu K, Ushio Y, et al. Meningeal gliomatosis models as a chemosensitivity assay system. Gan To Kagaku Ryoho 1984; 11:458-463.
11. Yoshida T, Shimizu K, Ushio Y, et al. Development of experimental meningeal gliomatosis models in rats. J Neurosurg 1986; 65:503-7.
12. Yoshida T, Shimizu K, Ushio Y, et al. Treatment of a rat meningeal gliomatosis model with neocarzinostatin. No To Shinkei 1987; 39:615-9.
13. Yoshida T, Shimizu K, Koulousakis A, Strum V. Intrathecal chemotherapy with ACNU in a meningeal gliomatosis rat model. J Neurosurg 1992; 77:778-782.
14. Herrlinger U, Buchholz R, Jachimczak P, Schabet M. Intrathecal treatment of C6 glioma leptomeningeal metastatis in Wistar rats with interleukin-2. J Neurooncol 1996; 27:193-203.
15. Kooistra KL, Rodriguez M, Powis G, et al. Development of experimental models of meningeal neoplasia using intrathecal injection of 9L gliosarcoma and walker 256 carcinosarcoma in the rat. Cancer Res 1986; 46:317-23.
16. Rewers AB, Redgate ES, Deutsch M, Fisher ER, Boges SS. A new rat brain tumor model: glioma disseminated via the cerebral spinal fluid pathways. J Neurooncol 1990; 8:213-19.
17. Ram Z, Walbridge S, Oshiro EM, et al. Intrathecal gene therapy for malignant leptomeningeal neoplasia. Cancer Res 1994; 54:2141-5.
18. Kramm CM, Rainov NG, Sena-Esteves M, et al. Herpes vector-mediated delivery of marker genes to disseminated central nervous system tumors. Hum Gene Ther 1996; 7:291-300.
19. Kramm CM, Rainov NG, Sena-Esteves M, et al. Long-term survival in a rodent model of disseminated brain tumors by combined intrathecal delivery of herpes vectors and ganciclovir treatment. Hum Gene Ther 1996; 7:1989-94.
20. Vincent AJ, Esandi MD, van Someren G, et al. Treatment of leptomeningeal metastases in a rat model using a recombinant adenovirus containing the HSV-tk gene. J Neurosurg 1996; 85:648-54.
21. Kramm CM, Chase M, Herrlinger U, et al. Therapeutic efficiency and safety of a second-generation replication-conditional HSV1 vector for brain tumor gene therapy. Hum Gene Ther 1997; 8:2057-68.
22. Sahu SK, Wen PY, Foulon CF, et al. Intrathecal 5-[125I]iodo-2'-deoxyuridine in a rat model of leptomeningeal matastases. J nucl Med 1997; 38:386-90.
23. Ushio Y, Posner JB, Shapiro WR. Chemotherapy of experimental meningeal carcinomatosis. Cancer Res 1977; 37:1232-7.
24. Ushio Y, Shimizu K, Aragaki Y, et al. Alteration of blood-CSF barrier by tumor invasion into the meninges. Neurosurgery 1981; 55:445-9.
25. Shimizu K, Ushio Y, Hayakawa T, Mogami H. Combination chemotherapy with 1-(4-amino-2-methyl-5-pyrimidinyl)-methyl-3-(2-chloroethyl)-3-nitrosurea hydrochloride and bleomycin in meningeal carcinomatosis in the rat. Can Res 1980; 40:1341-3
26. Kooistra KL, Rodriguiz M, Powis G. Toxicity of intrathecally administered cytotoxic drugs and their antitumor activity against an intrathecal Walker256 carcinosarcoma model for meningeal carcinomatosis in the rat. Cancer Res 1989; 49:977-82.
27. Jamshidi J, Yoshimine T, Ushio Y, et al. Pathology of brain parenchyma in meningeal carcinomatosis; immunohistochemical study with astroprotein (GFAP) and tubulin. J Neurooncol 1987; 5:65-71.
28. Izumoto S, Arita N, Ushio Y, Hayakawa T, et al. Growth activity of meningeal carcinomatosis—immunohistochemical study using anti-BrdU monoclonal antibody. No To Shinkei 1988; 40:127-31.
29. Hiesiger EM, Picco Del-Bo A, Lipschutz et al. Experimental meningeal carcinomatosis selectivity depresses local cerebral glucose utilization in rat brain. Neurology 1989; 39:90-5.

30. Huang TY, Howng SL. Intrathecal ACNU against experimental leptomeningeal tumors. Kao Hsiung I Hsueh Ko Hsueh Tsa Chih 1997; 13:626-30.
31. Huang TY, Hwang SL, Howng SL. Immunohistochemical demonstration with anti-bromodeoxyuridine monoclonal antibody in experimental meningeal carcinomatosis model. Kao Hsiung I Hsueh Tsa Chih 1997; 13:136-40.
32. Verinois FD, Wu JK, Qi P, Cano WG, Van Cherington. Tumor cells expressing the herpes simplex virus-thymidine kinase gene in the treatment of Walker256 meningeal neoplasia in rats. J Neurosurg 1996; 84:250-7.
33. Sagar SM, Price KJ. An experimental model of leptomeningeal metastases employing rat mammary carcinoma cells. J Neurooncol 1995; 23:15-21.
34. Miree J, Harwood TR, Gold S. The implantation of V-2 carcinoma in the subarachnoid space of rabbits. J Natl Med Assoc 1973;64:305-7.
35. Miree J, Gold S. Relationship of survival with number of V-2 carcinoma cells implanted in the subrachnoid space of rabbits. J Natl Med Assoc 1973; 65:407-9.
36. Frank JA, Girton M, Dwyer AJ, et al. Meningeal carcinomatosis in the VX-2 rabbit tumor model: Detection with Gd-DTPA-enhanced MR Imaging. Radiol 1988; 167:825-9.
37. Phillips PC, Than TT, Cork LC, et al. Intrathecal 4-hudroperoxycyclophosphamide: neurotoxicity, cerebrospinal fluid pharmacokinetics, and antitumor activity in a rabbit model of VX2 leptomeningeal carcinomatosis. Cancer Res 1992; 52:6168-74.
38. Miner KM, Kawaguchi T, Uba GW, Nicholson GL. Clonal drift of cell surfaces, melanogeneic, and experimental metastatic properties of in vivo-selected, brain meninges-colonizing murine B16 melanoma. Cancer Res 1982; 42:4631-8.
39. Siegal T, Sandbank U, Gabizon A, et al. Alteration of blood-brain-CSF barrier in experimental meningeal carcinomatosis. A morphologic and adriamycin-penetration study. J Neurooncol 1987; 4:233-42.
40. Thomas LB, Chirigos MA, Humphreys SR, Goldin A. Pathology of the spread of L1210 leukemia in the central nervous system of mice and the effect of treatment with cytoxan. J Natl Cancer Inst 1962; 28:1355-89.
41. Thomas LB, Chirigos MA, Humphreys SR, Goldin A. Developmant of meningeal leukemia (L1210) during treatment of subcutaneously inoculated mice with methotrexate. Cancer 1964; 17:352-60.
42. Chirigos MA, Thomas LB, Humphreys SR, Glynn JP, Goldin A. Therapeutic and immunological response of mice with meningeal leukemia (L1210) to challenge with an antifolic-resistant variant. Cancer Res 1964; 24:409-15.
43. Chirigos MA, Humphreys SR. Effect of alkylating agents on meningeal leukemia L1210 arising in methotrexate-treated mice. Cancer Res 1966; 26:1673-7.
44. Lynch RG, Medoff G, Valeriote F. A murine model for central nervous system leukemia and its possible relevance to human leukemia. J Natl Cancer Inst 1975; 55:611-7.
45. Fiebig HH, Zeller WJ, Schmähl D. An experimental model for meningeal leukemia in rats (L5222). Effect of treatment with BCNU and cyclophosphamide. Int J Cancer 1976; 18:710-6.
46. Varakis JN, Kase CS, Wilborn WH, Cheshire LB, Peterson RDA. Pathogenesis of an experimental meningeal leukemia model. Clin Immunol Immunopathol 1982; 23:400-7
47. Suzuki M, Abe I, Sato H. Changes in drug delivery (by blood-brain barrier dysfunction) on arachnoid leukemia: implication for CNS leukemic dissemination. Clin Exp Metastasis 1983; 1:163-71.
48. Hoogerbrugge PM, Hagenbeek A. Leptomeningeal infiltration in the rat models for acute myelocytic and lymphocyttic leukemia. Leukemia Res 1985; 9:1397-404.
49. Urch CE, George AJ, Stevenson GT, et al. Intra-thecal treatment of leptomeningeal lymphoma with immunotoxin. Int J Cancer 1991; 47:909-15.

50. Zovickian J, Youle RJ. Efficacy of intrathecal immunotoxin therapy in an animal model of leptomeningeal neoplasia. J Neurosurg 1988; 68:767-74.
51. Perk K, Pearson JW, Torgensen JA, Chirigos MA. An animal model for meningeal leukemia. Int J Cancer 1974; 13:863-6.
52. Peterson RDA, Varakis JN, Cheshire LB. New experimental model of meningeal leukemia. Cancer Res 1980; 40:3130-3.
53. Kupper H, Gerlach H, Wessel H, et al. Involvement of the central nervous system in malignant lymphomas of mice. Exp Pathol 1987; 31:185-9.
54. Siegal T, Okon E, Levy E, Mizrachi R, Hochman J. Introduction of adherent variants into the subarachnoid space (SAS) potentiates immune response protection to a syngeneic malignant lymphoma. Neurology 1986; 36(Suppl):187.
55. Yoshida T, Shimizu K, Ushio Y, et al. Development of experimental meningeal gliomatosis models using nude mice. Gan To Kagaku Ryoho 1986; 13:2745-50.
56. Miyao Y, Shimizu K, Okamoto Y, et al. Meningeal gliomatosis model in nude mice. Gan To Kagaku Ryoho 1986; 13:2600-5.
57. Miyao Y, Shimizu K, Okamoto Y, et al. Antitumor efficacy of recombinant interferon-beta on human gliomas. Gan To Kagaku Ryoho 1987; 14:490-4.
58. Abernathey CD, Kooistra KL, Wilcox GL, Laws ER Jr. New xenograft model for assessing experimental therapy of central nervous system tumors: human glioblastoma in the intrathecal compartment of the nude mouse. Neurosurgery 1988; 22:877-81.
59. Yamashita Y, Takahashi H, Nakazawa S. Experimental study on immunotherapy of meningeal gliomatosis with monoclonal antibody. No To Shinkei 1993; 45:63-70.
60. Fuchs HE, Archer GE, Colvin OM, et al. Activity of intrathecal 4-hydroperoxycyclophosphamide in a nude rat model of neuroplastic meningitis. Cancer Res 1990; 50:1954-9.
61. Friedman HS, Archer GE, McLendon RE,et al. Intrathecal melphalan therapy of human neoplastic meningitis in athymic nude rats. Cancer Res 1994; 54:4710-4.
62. Bergman I, Ahdab-Barmada M, Kemp SS, Griffen JA, Cheung NK. A rat model of leptomeningeal human neuroplastic xenografts. J Neurooncol 1997; 34:221-31.
63. Yamada M, Shimizu K, Tamura K, et al. Murine model of leptomeningeal dessimination using human medulloblastoma cells. Neurol Med Chir (Tokyo) 1991; 31:763-7.
64. Schabet M, Buchholz R, Schuster M, Pietsch T. Animal model of human medulloblastoma: clinical magnetic resonance imaging and histopathological findings. Med Ped Oncol 1997; 29:92-7.
65. Rosenfeld MR, Bergman I, Schramm L, et al. Adeno-associated viral vector gene transfer into leptomeningeal xenografts. J Neurooncol 1997; 34:139-44.
66. Myklebust AT, Godal A, Fodstad O. Targeted therapy with immunotoxins in a nude rat model for leptomeningeal growth of human small cell lung cancer. Cancer Res 1994; 54:2146-50.
67. Myklebust AT, Helseth A, Breistøl K, Hall WA, Fodstad O. nude rat models for human tumor metastases to CNS. Procedures for intracarotid delivery of cancer cells and drugs. J Neurooncol 1994; 21:215-24.
68. Pastan IH, Archer GE, McLendon RE, et al. Intrathecal administration of single-chain immunotoxin, LMB:7 [B3(Fv)-PE38], produces cures of carcinomatous meningitis in a rat model. Proc Natl Acad Sci 1995; 92:2765-9.
69. Schabet M, Wiethölter H, Meier D. Experimental meningeal neoplasia in nude rats. Neurology 1987; 37:311.
70. Schabet M, Ohneseit P, Buchholz R, Santo-Holtje L, Schmidberger H. Intrathecal ACNU treatment of leptomeningeal metastasis in a new athymic rat model. J Neurooncol 1992; 14:169-75.

71. Schabet M, Ohneseit P, Herrlinger U, Buchholz R. Intrathecal treatment of B16-F10 melanoma leptomeningeal metastases (LM) in nude rats with MTX, ACNU, or the combination of IFN-gamma and TNF-alpha. Brain Pathol 1994; 4:436.
72. Martos J, Petersen D, Klose U, et al. MR imaging of experimental meningeal melanomatosis in nude rats. J Neurooncol 1992; 14:207-11.
73. Herrlinger U, Schabet M, Buchholz R, Pietsch T. Leptomeningeal metastasis in the nude rat after intracisternal application of murine or human tumor cells. Brain Pathol 1994; 4:445.
74. Hall WA, Myklebust A, Godal A, Nesland JM, Fodstad Ö. In vivo efficacy of intrathecal tranferrin-pseudomonas exotoxin A immunotoxin against LOX melanoma. Neurosurgery 1994; 34:649-56.
75. Reijneveld JC, Taphoorn MJ, Voest EE. A simple mouse model for leptomeningeal metastases and repeated intrathecal therapy. J Neurooncol 1999; 42:137-42.
76. Zalutsky MR, McLendon RE, Garg PK, et al. Radioimmunotherapy of neoplastic meningitis in rats using an *-particle-emiting immunoconjugate. Cancer Res 1994; 54:4719-25.
77. Kobayashi T. New developments in chemotherapy for experimental brain metastasis. Gan To Kagaku Ryoho 1985; 12(3 Pt 2):757-65.
78. Cavallo F, Forni M, Riccardi C, et al. Growth and spread of human malignant T lymphoblasts in immunosuppressed nude mice: a model for meningeal leukemia. Blood 1992; 80:1279-83.
79. Herrlinger U, Schabet M, Schuster M, et al. Intracisternal treatment of CEM T-cell lymphoma leptomeningeal metastasis in nude rats with intracisternal ricin A-coupled anti-CD7 immunetoxin. Clin Neuropathol 1995; 14:264.
80. Breistøl K, Balzarini J, Sandvold ML, et al. Antitumor activity of P-4055 (elaidic acid-cytarabine) compared to cytarabine in metastatic and s.c. human tumor xenograft models. Cancer Res 1999; 59:2944-9.
81. Epstein AL, Herman MM, Kim H, Dorfman RF, Kaplan HS. Biology of the human malignant lymphomas. III. Intracranial heterotransplantation on the nude, athymic mouse. Cancer 1976; 37:2158-76.
82. Pinkel D, Woo S. Prevention and treatment of meningeal leukemia in children. Blood 1994; 84:355-66.
83. Wasserstrom WR, Glass JP, Posner JB. Diagnosis and treatment of leptomeningeal metastases from solid tumors. Cancer 1982; 49:759-772.
84. Chamberlain MC. Current concepts in leptomeningeal metastasis. Curr Opinion Oncol 1992; 4:533-539.
85. Steinherz PG. CNS leukemia: problem of diagnosis, treatment, and outcome. J Clin Oncol 1995; 13:310-3.
86. Herrlinger U, Weller M, Schabet M. New aspects of immunotherapy of leptomeningeal metastasis. J Neurooncol 1998; 38:233-9.
87. Zovickian J, Youle RJ. Efficacy of intrathecal immunotoxin therapy in an animal model of leptomeningeal neoplasia. J Neurosurg 1988; 68:767-74.
88. Herrlinger U, Schmidberger H, Buchholz R, et al. Intrathecal therapy of leptomeningeal CEM T-cell lymphoma in nude rats with anti-CD7 ricin toxin A chain immunotoxin. J Neurooncol 1997; 40:1-9.
89. Vrionis FD, Wu JK, Qi P, Cano WG, Cherington V. Tumor cells expressing the herpes simplex virus-thymidine kinase gene in the treatment of Walker 256 meningeal neoplasia in rats. J Neurosurg 1996; 84:250-7.
90. Schabet M, Herrlinger U. Animal models of leptomeningeal metastasis. J Neurooncol 1998; 38:199-205.

Chapter 11

IMPROVING THE OUTCOME OF PATIENTS WITH LEPTOMENINGEAL CANCER: NEW CLINICAL TRIALS AND EXPERIMENTAL THERAPIES

Kurt A. Jaeckle, M.D.
Mayo Clinic, Jacksonville, Florida 32224

Abstract: Current therapy for leptomeningeal metastases is predominantly palliative. In an effort to improve disease control and patient outcome, new strategies are being developed to target the cerebrospinal space. These include new intrathecal formulations of systemic chemotherapy as well as the development of radiolabeled immunoconjugates and antitumor antibodies. Furthermore, there is debate as to the optimal strategy of drug delivery for leptomeningeal tumor.

Key Words: Leptomeningeal metastases, clinical trials, systemic chemotherapy, immunoconjugates, radioisotopes

1. INTRODUCTION

Despite over 50 years of clinical experience in treating neoplastic meningitis, few effective therapies have been identified. Although one reason for this failure is the lack of effective agents, there are many additional obstacles.

Many intrathecal (IT) chemotherapeutic agents currently in use are cell-cycle specific, which potentially limits their efficacy in this particular disease setting. Prior studies have reported that cycling of cerebrospinal fluid (CSF) tumor cells is relatively slow, with only 55% of tumor cells cycling in a 10 day span. Most CSF tumor cells appear to be in G_0, with approximately 0.1% in S phase, and 1% in mitosis.[1,2] Unfortunately, the half-life of many intrathecal agents is measured only in minutes, as with thio-TEPA, mafosfamide, diaziquone, topotecan, and carmustine (BCNU); or in a few hours, as for cytarabine and methotrexate (MTX).

Tumor exposure is also affected by the limited penetration of intrathecal agents through the typically thickened membranes and tumor nodules. The depth of drug penetration appears relatively limited even in normal brain tissues. Blasberg reported his results in Rhesus monkeys given intrathecal MTX, cytarabine, thio-TEPA, and BCNU by ventriculocisternal perfusion.[3] At 1 hour of steady state perfusion, none of the drugs achieved concentrations greater than 1% of the CSF drug levels at distances 3.2 mm or greater from the ependymal surface.

The problem is further complicated by regional inhomogeneity of CSF flow. CSF drug distribution can be erratic due to irregular infiltration of the meninges by tumor cells, with resultant fibrosis and adhesions, in particular around the basal cisterns and distal lumbar thecal sac.[4]

Finally, patients commonly develop neoplastic meningitis in the setting of advanced systemic or central nervous system (CNS) metastases, which have often been resistant to prior radiation and chemotherapy. In addition, many of the histologic subtypes that commonly produce neoplastic meningitis are considered relatively resistant to therapy. When considering all these issues as a whole, it is not surprising why treatment often fails.

2. 'STANDARD' TREATMENTS FOR NEOPLASTIC MENINGITIS

There are several unresolved controversial issues with respect to treatment of patients with neoplastic meningitis (Table 1).

Table 1. Unresolved Controversies in Treatment of Neoplastic Meningitis

Intrathecal vs. intraventricular therapy
Systemic vs. intrathecal therapy
Multiagent vs. single agent intrathecal therapy
Role of combined systemic and intrathecal therapy
Role of radiotherapy
Identification of responsive histologic subgroups
Optimal timing of therapy
Role of prophylaxis in high risk histologies
Role of maintenance in responding patients

These issues must be addressed through the conduct of carefully designed, prospective clinical trials. To date there are no 'standard' treatments for neoplastic meningitis that have been shown to prolong overall survival of patients with neoplastic meningitis in controlled, prospective randomized trials. However, by default, some chemotherapeutic agents with palliative benefit, as demonstrated in clinical trials have become community standards of care for highly selected patients. Radiotherapy to symptomatic sites of disease has also produced palliative benefit and is considered a reasonable approach by most oncologists.

2.1 Intrathecal chemotherapy

Several chemotherapeutic agents have been administered intrathecally, including MTX, thio-TEPA, cytarabine (ara-C), BCNU, 3-[4-amino-2-methyl-5-pyrimidinyl)methyl]-1-nitrosourea hydrochloride (ACNU), and diaziquone (AZQ). These agents have largely produced dissatisfying results, but occasional anecdotal responders or long term survivors have been reported. To date, the four intrathecal agents that have been utilized most often in clinical practice in the United States are MTX, ara-C, sustained release ara-C, and thio-TEPA. There is also increasing enthusiasm for the use of high-dose systemic MTX (e.g., greater than 3 grams/m^2) as an alternative to intrathecal therapy. Although activity of these agents has been demonstrated, none have unequivocally prolonged survival in patients with neoplastic meningitis.

Combination therapy with intrathecal agents has also been attempted with conflicting results. A trial of intrathecal MTX, thioTEPA and cortisone on Day 1 followed by intrathecal cytarabine, MTX and hydrocortisone on Day 5 weekly in 13 breast cancer patients, with concomitant systemic chemotherapy and whole brain radiotherapy in 7 patients, failed to produce objective responses or improve symptoms.[5] However, a comparison of single agent intrathecal MTX (N=29) to a three drug regimen of MTX, cytarabine, and hydrocortisone (N=26) administered twice a week to solid tumor neoplastic meningitis patients showed a higher incidence of cytologic response (38.5% Vs 13.8%, p=0.036) and median survival (18.6 wk Vs 10.4 wk, p=0.029) in the combination therapy arm versus the single agent arm.[6]

2.2 Sustained-release and infusional intrathecal chemotherapy

As mentioned previously, most available intrathecal agents have short pharmacologic half-lives (T ½), which limit their efficacy. Prolonged drug exposure has been forwarded as a method to increase the cytotoxicity of such agents in CSF. It has been shown that some cell lines may be resistant in short exposure conditions, but demonstrate sensitivity with prolonged exposure. For example, in the human SO-M19 melanoma line, there was no inhibition of tritiated thymidine incorporation with short (2 hour) exposures despite concentrations of up to 4 ug / ml ara-C, whereas low concentrations (1 ug / ml) over a longer duration of 48 hours produced 90% inhibition of thymidine incorporation.[7]

Investigators have also explored continuous CSF drug administration in the treatment of neoplastic meningitis. In clinical trials, continuous ventriculocisternal or ventriculolumbar infusion of BCNU, and ACNU have been attempted.[8] These studies showed feasibility and relative safety of these procedures in experienced hands with suggestions of palliative effects.

Another approach to increasing duration of drug exposure involves the use of sustained release formulations. Hybrid liposomes with encapsulated BCNU have been administered intrathecally in meningeal gliomatosis rat models (human U-105-MG, U-251-MG, U-373-MG, and rat C6 and 9L), extending the half-life in CSF, and producing modest improvements in survival over 'free' BCNU – treated animals.[9] A lipid-based encapsulated formulation of MTX has also been studied in a rat model, which prolonged the CSF T ½ to 5.4 days as compared with 0.30 days for unencapsulated MTX.

The largest experience to date with this approach has involved an extended release formulation of cytarabine. Intralumbar administration of sustained release cytarabine resulted in a T 1/2 of 277 hours,[10] as compared with 1.45 - 3.4 hours for non-encapsulated cytarabine.[11,12] A comparative phase III prospective, randomized trial of this agent in patients with neoplastic meningitis from solid tumors has been reported.[13] Sixty-one patients with histologically proven cancer and positive CSF cytology were randomized to receive IT sustained-release cytarabine (SR-ara-C) (31 patients) every two weeks for three months, or IT MTX (30 patients) on a twice weekly basis, followed by a gradual taper in frequency over three months. Responses occurred in 26% of SR-ara-C-treated and 20% of MTX-treated patients ($p = 0.76$). Median survival was 105 days in the SR-ara-C arm and 78 days in the MTX arm ($p = 0.15$). There was a statistically significant extension in time to neurological progression, which favored SR-ara-C over MTX (58 versus 30 days; $p = 0.007$), and longer neoplastic meningitis-specific median survival (343 versus 98 days; $p = 0.074$).

Another study reported the results following treatment with sustained-release cytarabine in 43 patients with carcinomatous meningitis from breast cancer.[14] Sustained release ara-C 50 mg was administered every two weeks for one month; responding patients were then given up to three months of consolidation therapy. The intent-to-treat response rate was 21% (CI 95%: 12-34%). Median time to neurologic progression was 49 days (range, 1-515+), median survival 88 days (range, 1-515+). The major adverse events were headache and transient arachnoiditis. Headache occurred on 11% of cycles; 90% were grade 1 or 2. Transient arachnoiditis occurred on 19% of cycles; 88% were grade 1 or 2.

Sustained release ara-C has been utilized in a phase III prospective trial in patients with lymphomatous meningitis.[15] Twenty-eight patients were randomized to receive SR-ara-C 50 mg once every two weeks or free ara-C 50 mg twice a week for one month. Responding patients received an additional three months of consolidation therapy and then four months of maintenance therapy. The response rate was 71% for SR-ara-C and 15% for ara-C on an intent-to-treat basis (P = 0.006). There were no significant differences in time to neurologic progression or survival; however, when comparing SR-ara-C to conventional ara-C (median, 78.5 Vs 42 days and 99.5 Vs 63 days, respectively; P >.05). The major adverse events on both arms were headache and transient arachnoiditis.

Finally, a clinical trial has been initiated which attempts to increase drug exposure or 'concentration times time' (C X T) by continuous infusion via subcutaneous mechanical pumps, similar to those used for administration of intrathecal opiates for pain management.

Although these approaches are quite promising, no increase in survival of neoplastic meningitis patients has been demonstrated by methods that increase the duration of drug concentration in CSF. Additional clinical experience is necessary, which must also define any potential detrimental neurotoxic or hematologic effects of continuous or prolonged CSF drug exposure.

2.3 Systemic chemotherapy

There is some evidence that one can produce adequate CSF levels with high dose systemic chemotherapy, at least in the setting of neoplastic meningitis. Cytotoxic levels of MTX can be achieved with systemic administration, although the typical CSF level of MTX is only 3% that of the serum concentration. Administration of high dose MTX (8 grams / M2 over 4 hours) in 16 patients resulted in peak concentrations of 3.7 - 55 uM / L in CSF. These levels were maintained longer than that observed following single IT dosing. Clearance of CSF tumor cells was noted in 81% of patients, with a prolongation of survival to 13.8 months as compared to 2.3 months in an intrathecal MTX control group.[16]

The pharmacokinetics and toxicity of high-dose intravenous MTX with leucovorin rescue has been further explored in patients with neoplastic meningitis (Tetef et al, 2000). Sixteen patients were treated with intravenous doses of MTX, initially 200 – 1500 mg / M^2 followed by 23 hour infusion of 800 – 6000 mg / M^2. The pharmacokinetic data was compared to that from three patients receiving high-dose MTX without neoplastic meningitis. These authors concluded that the MTX levels obtained in CSF were higher in patients with neoplastic meningitis, presumably due to increased blood brain barrier permeability resulting from inflammation. Cytotoxic concentrations of CSF MTX, at levels > 1 uM, were obtained with these systemic doses in all patients and the CSF MTX half-life was 8.7 ± 3.4 hours. Based on grade 3 hematologic toxicity, these authors suggested a loading dose of 700mg/M2 followed by a 23 hour infusion of 2800 mg/M2. However, no patient in their study had an objective response with this schedule.[17]

Siegal has raised the provocative question of whether IT therapy is necessary or beneficial at all.[18] In review of their data, elimination of IT chemotherapy did not result in a diminished survival of patients with neoplastic meningitis from solid tumors. Two separate groups of patients were studied; Group 1, representing 54 patients receiving radiotherapy, IT therapy, and systemic therapy; and Group 2, 50 patients treated with radiation and systemic chemotherapy with no IT treatment. This retrospective study was not case controlled, but groups were of similar age and distribution of cancer types. There was no difference in median survival between the two groups (four months); however, neurotoxicity was higher in the group that received IT therapy. This group concluded that exclusion of intra-CSF chemotherapy from the treatment does not change overall response or survival or the proportion of long-term survivors.[19] However, another way of interpreting this data is that the IT therapies utilized to date are simply ineffective. This does not preclude the future identification of effective therapies that would be administered by an IT approach.

3. NEWER INVESTIGATIONAL TREATMENTS

3.1 Intrathecal chemotherapy

3.1.1 Preclinical studies

Busulfan, an alkylating agent, has been prepared in a soluble microcrystalline formulation. Busulfan has been administered in a human glioma D-456MG rat neoplastic meningitis model. IT busulfan produced a 60% survival increase over rats treated with saline.[20] A clinical multi-center trial is now underway.

IT melphalan has also been utilized in a athymic rat model of TE671 human rhabdomyosarcoma and the D54-MG human glioma. This latter agent has increased the median survival of rats nearly 500% over controls in these two tumor models, and has been utilized in a phase I clinical trial.[21]

A solubilized microcrystalline preparation of temozolomide, a methylating agent, has also been utilized in an athymic rat neoplastic meningitis model of malignant glioma. Injections of four doses of IT temozolomide produced increases in median survival at several dose levels in both MER - positive (methyl-excision-repair) and MER - negative human malignant glioma xenografts. However, neurotoxicity (patchy demyelination) was noted in some animals at the highest doses tested.[22]

Two additional alkylating agents that have received attention include 4-hydroperoxycyclophosphamide (4-HC) and mafosfamide. 4-HC has shown activity in a nude rat model of TE671 and D54MG neoplastic meningitis. Mafosfamide is a deriviative of cyclophosphamide that does not require prior hepatic activation in order to exert its alkylating effect.

3.2 Clinical studies

A phase I trial involving 23 patients treated with intraventricular topotecan via Ommaya reservoir recommended a Phase II dose of .4 mg in patients $\geq$ 3 years of age. Arachnoiditis characterized by fever, nausea or vomiting, headache, and back pain was the dose limiting side effect; 6/23 assessable patients had prolonged disease stabilization or response.[23,24] A phase II study in 27 adults with neoplastic meningitis treated with topotecan 0.4 mg intrathecally twice weekly for six weeks, followed by a tapering schedule, produced a median time to progression of six weeks and median overall survival of 13 weeks. Five (16%) patients cleared CSF of malignant cells, and additional 9 (30%) showed minor response or stability.[25]

IT mafosfamide produced an increase in median survival of 20% over that of historical controls.[26,27] This agent has also been evaluated in pediatric patients.[23] An uncontrolled trial has been reported utilizing intraventricular mafosfamide (up to 20mg) and concurrent systemic therapy of choice to 26 children with a variety of disseminated brain tumors twice weekly until remission or failure. Seven of 13 evaluable patients showed clearing of CSF malignant cells; toxicities included headache, nausea and vomiting.[28]

Anecdotal efficacy has been reported with systemic capecitabine monotherapy in breast cancer with neoplastic meningitis[29,30] and with intrathecal gemcitibine in non-small cell lung cancer.[31]

3.3 Radioisotopes

3.3.1 Preclinical studies

The radioisotope 5-[125I] iodo-2-deoxyuridine (125-IUDR), a thymidine analog, was evaluated in a 9L rat gliosarcoma model.[32] Rats received a bolus injection of 125-IUDR (10uCi) five days after tumor cell implantation. There was prolongation of the median time to paralysis to 15 days as compared with 11 days in control-treated animals. Autoradiography demonstrated that normal spinal cord cells did not show significant uptake. In a separate study, continuous infusion over 2-6 days of 125-IUDR showed isotope uptake in 9L tumor cells at various stages following engraftment. Animals were followed by magnetic resonance imaging (MRI). 125-IUDR - treated animals survived significantly longer than 127-IUDR control animals, with a 10-20% cure rate observed in test animals[33]. The combination of IT radioisotope with chemotherapy has also been explored in a TE-671 human rhabdomyosarcoma meningitis model in rats[34]. The combination of MTX and 125-IUDR extended the endpoint (time to paralysis) to 45 days from 24 days observed with IT MTX alone

5-Fluoro-2-deoxyuridine (FUDR) has shown limited activity in several murine neoplastic meningitis models, including the Walker 256 carcinoma, MM46 breast carcinoma, and 203-glioma, with acceptable neurotoxicity.[35]

3.3.2 Clinical studies

Continuous IT 5-fluoro-2'deoxyuridine (FdUrd) has been administered to 25 patients using a balloon pump system, eight of whom also received whole brain radiotherapy. Weekly changes of the FdUrd solution was made whenever possible. Clinical improvement in headache and nausea was observed in all patients, and CSF response was observed in 15 patients. The mean survival of patients not receiving whole brain radiotherapy was 285 ± 39 days; no significant toxicity was stated to have occurred.[36]

3.4 Intrathecal immunoconjugates

3.4.1 Preclinical studies

Recent studies have explored the potential of compartmental administration of antibodies coupled to radioisotopes (including beta or alpha emitters), or toxins derived from plants or bacteria. These targeting methods take advantage of the selective binding of specific antibodies, F(ab')2 fragments, or cloned single chain antibodies or fragments to specific tumor antigens which are generally absent in normal tissues. Theoretically, the binding of antibodies to antigenic targets may increase the duration of exposure over that possible with free isotope or toxin, while decreasing the toxicity to normal tissues. Most investigations to date have involved pre-clinical studies in murine or rat models of neoplastic meningitis.

The efficacy of 3F8 (anti-GD2) murine IgG-monoclonal antibody was tested in the treatment of a melanoma (SK-MEL-1) and neuroblastoma (NMB7) in athymic rats.[37] Antibody was administered by continuous ventricular infusion with or without lipopolysaccharide (LPS). When administered after three days of tumor engraftment, brain tumor growth was prevented in 1/3 of SK-MEL-1 animals and 2/3 of NMB7 animals, but there was persistent growth in the spinal region. The combination of 3F8 plus LPS was superior to antibody alone or control- treated animals.

The identification of a mutated epidermal growth factor receptor in malignant gliomas (EGFRvIII), and subsequent generation of antibody specific for this receptor, has prompted a study of the potential therapeutic usefulness of this agent when bound to the Pseudomonas exotoxin (PE); this immunotoxin has been designated as MR-1. In athymic rats bearing U87deltaEGFR human gliomatous meningitis, prolongation of median survival to 600% over saline controls was noted after three sequential doses of MR-1.[38] The same group has studied another PE-conjugated monoclonal antibody, LMB-1, reactive with a carbohydrate epitope (B3) present on breast, lung and ovarian tumors. In a B3 antigen-positive A431 neoplastic meningitis athymic rat model, multiple doses increased the median survival from 9.5 days in saline control-treated animals to 40.5 days. There was no evidence of activity in neoplastic meningitis controls prepared with tumors that were B3 antigen negative.[39] Some animals displayed no evidence of subarachnoid neoplasm in post-mortem analysis.[40]

Preliminary evaluations of a transferrin - PE immunoconjugate in a melanoma model of neoplastic meningitis have also been promising.[41]

3.4.2 Clinical studies

Several small pilot and phase I clinical trials of immunoconjugates have been initiated. Although showing promise in early investigations, data regarding long term safety issues, particularly with respect to neurotoxicity, is generally lacking.

Preliminary investigation of the 131-I-Mel-14 F(ab')2 immunoconjugate has shown that antibody administration is feasible, and in a single case report, potentially efficacious.[42]

The largest experience to date with IT administration of radiolabeled antibodies has been performed in Bristol.[43] These investigators reported the treatment of 52 patients with neoplastic meningitis with 131-I-conjugated monoclonal antibodies with relative specificities for various tumor antigens. Radiolabeled antibodies (approximately 25-160 mCi) was administered by intraventricular or intralumbar approach in adult patients. Evidence of tumor localization was demonstrated in several patients by nuclear imaging techniques. The mean survival of responders was 39 months, versus four months in non-responders, in this uncontrolled trial. Fifty per cent of patients were alive beyond one year. Responses were seen most frequently in children with primitive neuro-ectodermal tumors (53%). Toxicity was mild, with no deaths felt attributable to treatment.

An 131-I-radiolabeled monoclonal antibody to the extracellular matrix protein tenascin (81C6 antibody), and an 131-I conjugated antibody to chondroitin proteoglycan sulfate (Mel-14), has produced CSF and radiographic responses in some patients[44].

3.5 Interferon and unconjugated monoclonal antibodies

A phase II trial of IT alpha interferon produced cytologic responses with stable clinical neurologic status in 10/22 (45%) patients with response duration of 8-40 weeks (median 16 weeks; toxicity included arachnoiditis in 60% of cycles and fatigue in most patients.[45]

The anti-CD20 antibody rituximab has been administered with reasonable tolerance in patients with relapsed CNS lymphoma.[46] Treatment with IT or intraventricular rituximab in single doses up to 35 mg was well tolerated in five out of six patients with primary CNS lymphoma and leptomeningeal lymphoma. One patient, however, developed acute neurotoxicity. CSF levels of rituximab were higher than observed with systemic administration. Clearing of CSF malignant cells was observed in four out of six patients, but parenchymal lesions did not respond.[47]

Trastuzumab, an antibody showing effectiveness in HER-2 positive metastatic breast cancer patients, has minimal penetration of the intact cerebral meninges. One study has even suggested that the incidence of metastatic CNS disease, including parenchymal and leptomeningeal metastases, may be increased in such patients receiving systemic trastuzumab. Of a study cohort of 122 patients with metastatic breast carcinoma without CNS metastases at initiation of trastuzumab treatment, 34% (95% C.I. 26, 44%) developed CNS metastases at a median of six months following initiation of treatment. Of these, 19% had leptomeningeal metastases; 50% of patients developing CNS metastases had stable or responding systemic metastatic disease.[48] These frequencies represent higher figures than historical controls (15-20% incidence of CNS metastases, and 6-8% incidence of leptomeningeal metastases in patients with breast cancer). Trials with IT trastuzumab have been initiated.[49]

3.5.1 Gene therapy

Transfection experiments have been attempted in order to alter and selectively target killing of CSF tumor cells. In feasibility studies, IT adeno-TK virus has successfully been administered to rats and non-human primates, and has been associated with an immune response, but also a certain degree of neurotoxicity.[50] Adenoviral transfer efficiency of the thymidine kinase-TK gene has been studied in a 9L gliosarcoma neoplastic meningitis model in rats. These studies have shown successful gene expression in the tumors, particularly when driven by a CMV gene promoter, with evidence of cytotoxicity following subsequent gancyclovir treatment. (Vincent et al, 1997) These are promising investigations that require further study.

4. SUMMARY AND CONCLUSIONS

Although treatment of neoplastic meningitis has been associated with poor response rates and has had minimal impact on overall survival, several promising new approaches that are under investigation will hopefully improve the prognosis for these patients. These include new chemotherapeutic agents, techniques that prolong drug exposure, targeted approaches, and gene therapy.

Since nearly three-quarters of patients with neoplastic meningitis die of complications of neoplastic meningitis, either alone or in combination with progressive systemic disease, any therapy with even marginal activity is likely to show benefit. However, successful new treatment strategies must surmount the known obstacles common to this interesting but devastating complication of cancer.

REFERENCES

1. Kuo AH, Yataganas X, Galicich JH, Fried J, Clarkson BD Proliferative kinetics of central nervous system (CNS) leukemia. Cancer 1975; 36:232-239.
2. Blasberg RG, Patlak CS, Shapiro WR. Distribution of methotrexate in the cerebrospinal fluid and brain after intraventricular administration. Cancer Treat Rep 1977; 61: 633-41.
3. Blasberg RG, Patlak C, Fenstermacher JD. Intrathecal Chemotherapy: Brain tissue profiles after ventriculocisternal perfusion. J Pharmacol Exp Ther 1975; 195: 73-83.
4. Chamberlain MC, Kormanik PA Prognostic significance of 111 indium – DTPA CSF flow studies in leptomeningeal metastases. Neurology 1996; 46:1674-7.
5. Orlando L, Curigliano G., Colleoni M., et al. Intrathecal chemotherapy in carcinomatous meningitis from breast cancer. Anticancer Res 2002; 22: 3057-59.
6. Kim DY, Lee KW, Yun T, et al. Comparison of intrathecal chemotherapy for leptomeningeal carcinomatosis of a solid tumor: methotrexate alone versus methotrexate in combination with cytosine arabinoside and hydrocortisone. Jpn J Clin Oncol 2003; 33:608-12.
7. Kern DH, Shoemaker RH, Hildebrand-Zanki SU, Driscoll JS Structure-activity relationships defining the cytotoxicity of catechol analogues against human malignant melanoma. Cancer Res 1988; 48:5178-82.
8. Kochi K, Kuratsu J, Mihara Y, Takaki et al. Ventriculolumbar perfusion of 3-[4-amino-2-methyl-5-pyrimidinylmethyl]-1-nitrosoureahydrochloride Neurosurg 1993; 33:817-23.
9. Kitamura, I, Kochi M, Matsumoto Y, Ueoka R, Kuratsu J, Ushio Y. Intrathecal chemotherapy with 1,3-bis(2-chloroethyl)-1-nitrosourea encapsulated into hybrid liposomes for meningeal gliomatosis: an experimental study. Cancer Res 1996; 56: 3986-82.
10. Chamberlain MC, Kormanik P, Kim S. Pharmacokinetics of intralumbar DTC-101 for the treatment of leptomeningeal metastases. Arch Neurol 1995; 52:912-7.
11. Esteva F.J, Soh LT, Holmes F.A., et al. Phase II trials and pharmacokinetic evaluation of cytosine arabinoside for leptomeningeal metastases form breast cancer. Cancer Chemother Pharmacol 2000; 46: 382-6.
12. Zimm S, Collins JM, Miser J, Chatter JID, Poplack DG. Cytosine arabinoside cerebrospinal fluid kinetics. Clin Pharmacol Ther 1984; 35:826-30.
13. Glantz MJ, Jaeckle KA, Chamberlain MC, et al. A randomized controlled trial comparing intrathecal sustained-release cytarabine (DepoCyt) to intrathecal methotrexate in patients with neoplastic meningitis from solid tumors. Clin Cancer Res 1999; 5:3349-51
14. Jaeckle KA, Phuphanich S, Bent MJ, et al. Intrathecal treatment of neoplastic meningitis due to breast cancer with a slow-release formulation of cytarabine. Br J Cancer 2001; 84:157-63.
15. Glantz MJ, LaFollette S, Jaeckle KA, et al. Randomized trial of a slow-release versus a standard formulation of cytarabine for the intrathecal treatment of lymphomatous meningitis. J

Clin Oncol 1999; 17:3110-6
16. Glantz MJ, Cole BF, Recht L, et al. High-dose intravenous methotrexate for patients with nonleukemic leptomeningeal cancer: is intrathecal chemotherapy necessary? J Clin Oncol 1998; 16:1561-7.
17. Tetef ML, Margolin KA, Doroshow JH, et al. Pharmacokinetics and toxicity of high-dose intravenous methotrexate in the treatment of leptomeningeal carcinomatosis Cancer Chemother Pharmacol. 2000; 46:19-26.
18. Siegal T. Leptomeningeal metastases: rationale for systemic chemotherapy or what is the role of intra-CSF chemotherapy? J Neuro Oncol 1998; 38:151-7.
19. Bokstein F, Lossos A, Siegal T. Leptomeningeal metastases from solid tumors: a comparison of two prospective series treated with and without intra-cerebrospinal fluid chemotherapy. Cancer 1998; 82:1756-63.
20. Archer GE, Sampson JH, McLendon RE, et al. Intrathecal busulfan treatment of human neoplastic meningitis in athymic nude rats. J Neuro Oncol 1999; 44:233-41.
21. Friedman H.S., Archer G.E., McLendon R.E., et al. Intrathecal melphalan therapy of human neoplastic meningitis in athymic nude rats. Cancer Res 1994; 54:4710-4.
22. Sampson JH, Archer GE, Villavicencio AT, et al. Treatment of neoplastic meningitis with intrathecal temozolomide. Clin Cancer Res 1999; 5:1183-8.
23. Blaney SM, Poplack DG: Neoplastic meningitis: diagnosis and treatment considerations. Med Oncol 2000; 17:151-62.
24. Blaney SM, Heideman R, Berg S, et al. Phase I clinical trial of intrathecal topotecan in patients with neoplastic meningitis. J Clin Oncol 2003; 21:243-7.
25. Groves MD, Baumgartner KE, Conrad CA,et al. A Phase II study of intrathecal topotecan in patients with meningeal malignancies. Neurology 2004; 62: 475(abstr.).
26. Fuchs HE, Archer GE, Colvin OM, et al. Activity of intrathecal 4-hydroperoxycyclophosphamide in a nude rat model of human neoplastic meningitis. Cancer Res 1990; 15:1954-9.
27. Slavc I, Schuller E, Czech T, Hainfellner JA, Seidl R, Dieckmann K. Intrathecal mafosfamide therapy for pediatric brain tumors with meningeal dissemination. J Neuro Oncol 1998; 38:213-8.
28. Slavc I, Schuller E, Falger J, et al. Feasibility of long-term intraventricular therapy with mafosfamide (n=26) and etoposide (n=11): experience in 26 children with disseminated malignant brain tumors. J Neurooncol 2003; 64:239-47.
29. Rogers LR, Remer SE, Tejwani S. Durable response of breast cancer leptomeningeal metastasis to capecitabine monotherapy. Neuro-oncol 2004; 6:63-4.
30. Giglio P, Tremont-Lukats IW, Groves MD. Response of neoplastic meningitis from solid tumors to oral capecitabine. J Neurooncol 2003; 65:167-72.
31. Chen YM, Chen MC, Tsai C.M, Perng RP. Intrathecal gemcitabine chemotherapy for non-small cell lung cancer patients with meningeal carcinomatosis-a case report. Lung Cancer 2003; 40:99-101.
32. Sahu SK, Wen PY, Foulon CF, et al. Intrathecal 5-[125I]iodo-2'-deoxyuridine in a rat model of leptomeningeal metastases. J Nucl Med 1997; 38:386-90.
33. Kassis AI, Wen PI, Van den Abbeele A.D, et al. 5-[125I] iodo-2-deoxyuridine in the radiotherapy of brain tumors in rats. J Nucl Med 1998; 39:1148-54.
34. Kassis AI, Dahman DA, Adelstein SJ. In-vivo therapy of neoplastic meningitis with methotrexate in 5-[125I] iodo-2-deoxyuridine (125 IUdR). Acta Oncol 2000; 39:731-7.
35. Nakagawa H, Yamada M, Fukushima M, Ikenaka K. Intrathecal 5-fluoro-2-deoxyuridine (FdUrd) for the treatment of solid tumor neoplastic meningitis: an in vivo study. Cancer Chemotherapy Pharmacol 1999; 43:247-56.

36. Nakagawa H, Tamura M, Fukushima S, Majima S. Continuous intrathecal chemotherapy with 5-fluoro-2'-deoxyuridine (FdUrd) in treatment of leptomeningeal carcinomatosis. Proc Am Soc Clin Oncol 2004; 23:123 (abstr).
37. Bergman I, Barmada MA, Heller G, Griffin JA, Chung MK. Treatment of neoplastic meningeal xenografts; intraventricular administration of an anti-ganglioside monoclonal antibody, 3F8. Int J Cancer. 1999; 12:538-48.
38. Archer GE, Sampson JH, Lorimer IA, et al. Regional treatment of epidermal growth factor vIII-expressing neoplastic meningitis with a single-chain immunotoxin MR-1. Clin Cancer Res 1999; 5:2646-52.
39. Bigner DD, Archer GE, McLendon RE, et al. Efficacy of compartmental administration of immunotoxin LMB-1 (B3-LysPE38) in a rat model of carcinomatous meningitis. Clin Cancer Res 1995; 1:1545-55.
40. Pastan IH, Archer GE, McLendon RE, et al. Intrathecal administration of single-chain immunotoxin, LMB-7 [B3(Fv)-PE38], produces cures of carcinomatous meningitis in a rat model. Proc Natl Acad Sci 1995; 28:2765-69.
41. Hall WA, Myklebust A, Godal A, Nesland JN, Fodstad O. In vivo efficacy of intrathecal transferrin-Pseudomonas exotoxin A immunotoxin against LOX melanoma. Neurosurgery 1994; 34: 649-55.
42. Cokgor I, Akabani G, Friedman HS, et al. Long term response in a patient with neoplastic meningitis secondary to melanoma treated with (131)I - radiolabeled antichondroitin proteoglycan sulfate Mel-14 F(ab')2: A case study. Cancer 2001; 91:1809-13.
43. Coakham HB, Kemshead JT. Treatment of neoplastic meningitis by targeted radiation using (131)I - radiolabeled monoclonal antibodies. Results of responses and long term follow-up in forty patients. J Neurooncol 1998; 38:225-32.
44. Bigner DD, Brown M, Coleman RE, et al. Phase I studies of treatment of malignant gliomas and neoplastic meningitis with 131-I- radiolabeled monoclonal antibodies anti-tenascin 81C6 and anti-chondroitin proteoglycan sulfate Mel-14 F(ab')2 - a preliminary report. J Neurooncol 1995; 24:109-22.
45. Chamberlain MC, A phase II trial of intra-cerebrospinal fluid alpha interferon in the treatment of neoplastic meningitis. Cancer 2002; 15:2675-80.
46. Schulz H., Pels H., Schmidt-Wolf I., Zeelen U., Germing U., Engert A. Intraventricular treatment of relapsed central nervous system lymphoma with the anti-CD20 antibody rituximab. Haematologica 2004; 89:753-4.
47. Schulz H, Pels H, Schlegel U, Zeelen U, Germing U, Engert A. Intraventricular application of rituximab as a treatment option in patients with CNS lymphoma and leptomeningeal disease. Proc Am Soc Clin Oncol 2004; 23:112 (abstr.)
48. Bendell JC, Domchek SM, Burstein H.J, et al. Central nervous system metastases in women who receive trastuzumab-based therapy for metastatic breast carcinoma. Cancer 2003; 15:2972-7.
49. Laufman LR, Forsthoefel KF. Use of intrathecal trastuzumab in a patient with carcinomatous meningitis. Clin Breast Cancer 2002; 2:316 (letter).
50. Driesse MJ, Esandi MC, Kros J.M, et al. Intra-CSF administered recombinant adenovirus causes an immune response-mediated toxicity. Gene Ther 2000; 7:1401-9.

Index